T0381556

7 Minutes
of Magic

7 Minutes of Magic

THE ULTIMATE ENERGY WORKOUT

Lee Holden
with Doug Abrams

AVERY
a member of
Penguin Group (USA) Inc.
New York

Published by the Penguin Group

Penguin Group (USA) Inc., 375 Hudson Street, New York, New York 10014, USA • Penguin Group (Canada), 90 Eglinton Avenue East, Suite 700, Toronto, Ontario M4P 2Y3, Canada (a division of Pearson Canada Inc.) • Penguin Books Ltd, 80 Strand, London WC2R 0RL, England • Penguin Ireland, 25 St Stephen's Green, Dublin 2, Ireland (a division of Penguin Books Ltd) • Penguin Group (Australia), 250 Camberwell Road, Camberwell, Victoria 3124, Australia (a division of Pearson Australia Group Pty Ltd) • Penguin Books India Pvt Ltd, 11 Community Centre, Panchsheel Park, New Delhi–110 017, India • Penguin Group (NZ), 67 Apollo Drive, Rosedale, North Shore 0632, New Zealand (a division of Pearson New Zealand Ltd) • Penguin Books (South Africa) (Pty) Ltd, 24 Sturdee Avenue, Rosebank, Johannesburg 2196, South Africa

Penguin Books Ltd, Registered Offices: 80 Strand, London WC2R 0RL, England

First trade paperback edition 2008
Copyright © 2007 by Lee Holden
Photographs copyright © 2007 by Kurt Kreutzer of Images Photography

The Library of Congress catalogued the hardcover as follows:

Holden, Lee.
7 minutes of magic : the ultimate energy workout / Lee Holden with Doug Abrams.
p.   cm.
Includes index.
ISBN 978-1-58333-276-4
1. Exercise.   2. Exercise—Physiological aspects.   3. Physical fitness.   I. Title.
RA781.H63   2007   2007003614
613.7—dc22

ISBN 978-1-58333-315-0 (paperback edition)

Book design by Mauna Eichner and Lee Fukui

Neither the publisher nor the authors are engaged in rendering professional advice or services to the individual reader. The ideas, procedures, and suggestions contained in this book are not intended as a substitute for consulting with a physician. All matters regarding health require medical supervision. Neither the authors nor the publisher shall be liable or responsible for any loss or damage allegedly arising from any information or suggestion in this book.

While the authors have made every effort to provide accurate telephone numbers and Internet addresses at the time of publication, neither the publisher nor the authors assume any responsibility for errors, or for changes that occur after publication. Further, the publisher does not have any control over and does not assume any responsibility for author or third-party websites or their content.

146122990

Contents

PART I

7 Minutes to Change Your Life

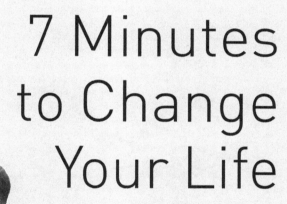

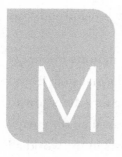odern life leaves us always on the run. Juggling the pressures of work and money, family and friends, often leaves us little time to take care of our health and well-being. I've developed 7 Minutes of Magic as a mind-body wellness program to dramatically improve your life in an amount of time that you can find in even your most hectic day.

Just how long is seven minutes? Putting it into perspective, most of us spend seven to eight hours sleeping, two to three hours making and eating meals, three to four hours watching television, and eight or more hours working. Is committing to a brief, seven-minute routine worth the effort if it means more energy and less stress in your daily life? Is it really that hard to find a seven-minute block of time to rejuvenate, recharge, and reinvigorate your mind and body? Look at it this way—there are seven minutes of commercials in a half-hour television sitcom. If you have to, you can do your 7 Minutes of Magic two or three minutes at a time during the commercials. It's not ideal, but it will still work. This book is about taking away the excuses so you can be healthy and full of energy.

In order to live a balanced life, you need two distinct kinds of energy: one to fire you up in the morning and the other to calm you down in the evening. As you will discover for yourself, the 7-minute morning routine is faster than waiting in line at Starbucks and will give you more energy and vitality throughout your day than a double latte—without the caffeine crash. In addition, you will find that the 7-minute evening routine is more relaxing than sipping a cocktail and will help you unwind and clear stress from the day—without the hangover.

Life today demands seemingly endless amounts of energy and all too often we are left feeling drained and exhausted. Everyone needs more energy, but most people have forgotten how to access it. This program will show you how to awaken the energy in your body and harness the energy that exists in the world all around you.

Energy Is True Magic

The word *magic* in this book has nothing to do with pulling rabbits from hats or the use of charms and spells. It is the word people who have learned these flowing routines use to describe the changes they experience in their bodies and minds—more energy, greater health, and less stress. Let me explain how this seemingly magical transformation occurs.

Within each of us there is a place that is full of energy, health, and happiness. This is our natural state, but we so often lose touch with it in our busy, distracted lives. A visit to this place of inner vitality and harmony every day, even for a brief seven minutes, allows us to access a higher level of energy, strengthen our immune systems, and transform the patterns and assumptions that limit our bodies and minds.

By clearing physical and mental stress every day, the body finds its natural state of balance. Stress compromises the immune system; exercise, deep breathing, and flowing movements strengthen it.

Real magic is not external; it is about an inner transformation and alchemy. You will learn to change the leaden, lethargic, low-energy state that so many of us experience when we wake up or return from a day of work into the golden, abundant, high-energy state that everyone craves and needs for true well-being.

Our habits shape the outcome of our lives, both internally and externally. To lead healthier, happier lives we need routines that support that outcome. Our bodies, like nature, grow from the inside out. To cultivate greater levels of energy and strength, the body needs consistent growth in that direction. A little bit every day—just seven minutes—is better than a lot once in a while.

Seven truly is a magic number. Modern psychology has shown that seven is the number of things that most people can remember—this is the reason that telephone numbers are generally limited to seven numbers. I've designed both the morning and evening routines as seven flows that anyone can remember and do, regardless of their age, body type, or level of fitness. The word *flow* is used to describe the exercises because one movement or stretch is followed by another, like moving water, so each routine is a seamless extension of the one that precedes it.

Seven minutes is the minimum amount of time needed to make changes in the body and mind that will have a lasting effect throughout the day. Think of boiling water—a certain amount of time is needed to reach a new state, to change from water into steam. For our bodies and minds, seven minutes is the amount of time needed to harness our energy to a new and healthier state. Doing seven flows in seven minutes allows us to absorb and integrate the benefits of the routines into our bodies and minds most efficiently.

This book draws on the principles and practices of ancient mind-body traditions, but presents them in a fluid and efficient routine for maximum benefit in minimal time. As you will see in the next section, both the morning and evening exercise programs are designed to match the rhythms of our bodies and the rhythms of nature.

A Lightning Flash of Vitality to Start Your Day

The morning is a particularly important time. How you start each day is crucial. Your mood and attitude during the first part of the day set the tone for the rest of what will follow. The morning routine presented in this book is designed to tap into the rising energy of the day. It allows you to sync your inner rhythm with the larger rhythm of nature, giving you greater energy, enthusiasm, and focus for the rest of the day.

Starting the day off right involves two essential ingredients. First is proper movement. After a long night of inactivity you need to fill the body with energy, or as the ancients said, you need to give yourself a "lightning flash of vitality." The 7-minute morning routine is designed to give you this rejuvenating flash.

The second ingredient is proper intent. By harmonizing the body and mind, we begin the day centered and focused. This is accomplished in the morning routine by first charging the body with energy and then finishing with a short visualization in a posture called Bamboo in the Wind (see page 79) to focus intent and create the day that we want to have.

Ending Your Day with Relaxation and a Good Night's Sleep

The evening, an equally important time, requires a completely different kind of energy. At this time we let go of the busy energy of the day and then fill up with a more relaxed and tranquil energy.

The evening routine is a quick way to release the stress and tension and get centered for life at home. Whether you have children to watch, dinner to prepare, or evening activities, this routine will help refresh and relax you as the day comes to a close. We don't usually have time for a bubble bath and a massage at the end of each day, but we do have seven minutes, and the evening routine can take us to a similar place of tranquility and balance so that we can enjoy our evening.

My goal in sharing this program is to give you a powerful and enduring routine that you can do in a short amount of time—no matter what other pressures and commitments you might have in your life. I want you to be able to wake up in the morning and charge up your mind and body to begin the day stronger, more energized, and more focused. I also want to help you end the day joyfully, clear stress and tension, and be able to truly let go and unwind for a better night's sleep. Then, as you sleep, your body can restore its energy so you can wake up even more refreshed and revitalized.

Before you learn the routines, I want you to know a little about the many traditions and techniques that come together in

7 Minutes of Magic and how they transformed my life. Then you will see how East and West, ancient traditions and modern fitness, come together to create a powerful and effective practice. I hope that knowing this background will enrich your practice and help you to understand the many levels—body, mind, and spirit—at which these practices can make a difference in your life journey. However, if all you have today is seven minutes, feel free to skip ahead to the flowing routines themselves!

1

My Story: Discovering Ancient Secrets for Modern Life

During college my greatest teachers were not professors, and the greatest lessons were not revealed in the classroom. I attended the University of California at Berkeley, which was home to more than twenty Nobel Prize–winning teachers, had an unprecedented research reputation, and was the number-one public university in the country. But the wisdom I acquired while I was in college came from teachers without Ph.D.'s who taught in a small building across town that I never would have known existed if I had not been led there.

When I arrived on campus my freshman year, I had no idea what lay ahead and was just trying, like the thousands of other students, to handle the newfound freedoms that I had living away from the watchful eyes of my parents for the first time. I quickly realized that smart, disciplined high school students can go a little overboard when finally let loose—and I was no exception.

By my junior year, I was trying to complete my psychology degree, play Division I soccer, and maintain a full social calendar. Part of me was having the time of my life, yet another part was stressed out, unhappy, overstimulated, and yearning for something deeper and more meaningful. I knew that taking psychology classes and studying the behavior of rats in mazes was unlikely to reveal the secrets of happiness. My grades were starting to slip, I was sitting on the bench on the soccer team, and my girlfriend had just broken up with me. I had reached the ocean bottom of my college life: I had a choice to make—become a better swimmer, or drown in my self-pity.

It was about a week later that circumstances threw me a life preserver. As I was sitting in class as usual, I noticed a woman sitting a few seats away from me. To my surprise, she was not taking any notes. Imagine a room of four hundred students frantically scribbling, straining to write down every detail, while she just sat there, spine straight, hands folded, keenly observing the professor. I smiled with amazement and disbelief. How could you actually do that—go to class and not take notes? Berkeley was highly competitive and intellectually challenging. Students worked extremely hard to grasp the information. After a few weeks of watching her, I finally introduced myself.

After a brief conversation, I asked her how she managed to go through classes like statistics and industrial psychology without putting a pen to paper. Her answer was simple: "The Tao." I looked at her, cocking my head like a dog does when it hears a funny sound. What? She offered to escort me to a class at a local tai chi studio that gave lectures on Taoism, Zen, chi, and yoga. She explained that there was a common thread that linked all these disciplines and that they could be used for practical purposes, like remembering everything in a lecture without taking notes. She explained to me that before her training, she was a stress case, a B student at best. Now she was the picture of mental calm, getting straight A's, and feeling energized every day. It sounded too good to be true.

We walked into an ordinary looking house on the north side of campus, up in the hills, with a view of the San Francisco Bay. The living room was large and spacious with nothing but cushions on the floor. There were somewhere between twelve and fifteen students sitting in the room. The teacher, Master Sun, smiled as we walked in and sat down. He was bald, wore loose pants and a white T-shirt, and had warm, radiant eyes. The strange thing was that I didn't feel weird walking into this room, even with fifteen pairs of curious eyes on me. There was a tranquility and peacefulness about the space.

The class began with deep breathing exercises, progressed to vigorous stretching, and ended with flowing movements. Trying to hold some of these postures required tremendous abdominal strength and balance. I was sweating as if I was sprinting through a soccer game on a hot day. The flowing movements required a dexterity that I was completely unfamiliar with. I was not used to moving my body that slowly and coordinating all the movements from the center of my body. Yet by the end of class, my body felt completely different. My hands and arms were tingling, my head was light, as if all my thoughts were put to rest, and I could feel an inner power coursing through my veins.

After the class, Master Sun lectured on the mind. He said something that I still remember to this day: "There is much more to the mind than just thinking. When your mind is silent, the Universe surrenders." Maybe this was a clue as to how my classmate was able to get straight A's without taking notes.

During the off season of soccer, I trained diligently at the center. The students there were quite different from the university students; it wasn't about getting good grades or competition, it was about going deeper into oneself. I learned the classic 108 tai chi moves. I took yoga three times a week, and I learned to meditate. Looking back, these were the most important life skills I acquired in the five years I spent at Berkeley.

As Master Sun emphasized in every class, tai chi is the art of effortless power; by learning to go with the flow of life, the struggle ceases. Now, this sounded great in theory, but I really didn't believe it in my gut. My whole life, I had worked hard in both school and sports to succeed. Effort, tenacity, and perseverance were all principles I could count on to get me through. But the more I trained in tai chi, the more I was beginning to witness effortlessness in my own life. In fact, during the next season, my soccer playing was transformed. I went from mediocre to outstanding. My endurance, speed, agility, and focus were all dramatically different. It was weird, like I had grown another lung. Not only was I faster, but I could play much longer and with more stamina. The benefits extended beyond my athletic ability. I was getting better grades without any extra studying. I was still taking notes in class, but my focus was noticeably improved.

Master Sun went on to explain that tai chi, Zen, and yoga didn't give you something that wasn't there, but like a sculptor carving a statue out of rock, they could reveal an inner potential that was always present.

When I graduated from the university, I immediately set out for Asia to study these disciplines where they had originated. I went to northern Thailand to study with Master Mantak Chia. I had attended one of his workshops while he was in Berkeley, and was struck by the simplicity and the power of the exercises. Here was a practice that was easy to learn, yet had tremendous benefits. Master Chia talked of longevity, vitality, and how to achieve a passionate, spiritual relationship with your partner. Master Chia described how one could use spirituality in a practical way to enhance everyday life without having to renounce the material world, as many monks, priests, nuns and spiritual practitioners do. He emphasized how the health of the body, the state of the emotions, the quality of the mind, and cultivation of the spirit practice were all intricately connected.

I spent four years going back and forth between the United States and Thailand. During my third trip, I was asked to be chief editor for all of Master Chia's publications. This was a fantastic opportunity to study and work directly with one of the foremost modern-day masters of Eastern philosophy, tai chi, Taoist yoga, and meditation. I would soon find that I had to pass rigorous tests before I would be allowed to write each new chapter or book. Master Chia wanted to make sure that I embodied the practices and principles that I was writing about.

Working with such a revered master was an awe-inspiring experience. I remember the first day of my new assignment, waking up at 5:30 a.m. before the group lectures and class instruction. I walked from my room to Master Chia's house through the lush Thai palm trees and jungle orchids. The sky was just beginning to open with color, the deep violet of night giving way to streaks of bright orange light peeking into the horizon. As I walked, everything around me was a new experience. The tropical air was warm and thick. Even the sound of the birds was a mysterious melody, like listening to music in another language. Despite the beauty all around me, I was nervous.

I had no idea what to expect or what Master Chia expected from me. As I approached his door and lifted my hand to knock, I hesitated. What if he meant 5:30 p.m.? I stopped, leaving my outstretched fist frozen in the air. I stood there listening for at least a minute. No sound. Just then, a voice above me said, "Your monkey mind is already thinking too much." I jumped at the words. Master Chia was above me, stretching on his balcony. "Come up," he said, without looking down or breaking the flow of his movement.

For the next month, I would go to Master Chia's house and work out every day. We would train for about an hour and a half, practicing tai chi, qi gong, breathing exercises, and meditation techniques. I had heard of the gentle martial art of tai chi, but qi gong, an ancient energy and wellness practice, was completely new to me. I later learned that qi gong was the foundation of tai chi and many other forms of martial arts.

What I kept realizing again and again was that this practice was not new age fluff, but a body-mind-spirit science. Master Chia was showing me formulas that had been tested for the last four thousand years. He explained that these exercise and meditation routines were like a well-trodden path to the top of the mountain. If you practice them, you will reach the peak and enjoy the expanding vista of a clear mind and radiant health.

Getting this information firsthand was an incredible learning experience. But keeping up with Master Chia was no easy task. He slept only four or five hours a night and had the energy of a power plant. He explained to me that nature had an unlimited amount of energy and all we needed to do was be receptive to it. Here was a man in his late fifties who slept very little, who never got sick, who traveled to fifteen countries a year, who wrote sixteen books in five years, and who had developed the Tao Garden, the first holistic health center to incorporate fitness, organic nutrition, tai chi, qi gong, and meditation.

Master Chia expected the most from me and was not easy on his students. I remember one day during lunch, I asked him a question about the tai chi form. He replied, "Show me your form." I hesitated. There were over a hundred people in the dining hall. "Right now?" I asked, pleading with my voice to postpone his request. "Now."

I took a deep breath, brought my feet together, and began the form. When I stepped into the first posture, my legs were trembling with nervous tension. I felt like Elvis as my knees shook back and forth. I could feel everyone in the room watching me, happily eating their Pad Thai noodles while I was sweating through the form. As I continued, Master Chia got up from his chair and walked around me. He firmly slapped me on the back three or four times, and said, "More power here." I continued focusing my awareness on the lower back area called the "door of life." Master Chia then began to push on my shoulders and hips as I moved. I struggled to keep my balance and maintain my center. I stumbled a few times as he pushed, but kept moving through the form as best as I could. This went on for what seemed like an eternity. Finally he sat back down and said, "You only need to do the form one thousand times more." It was a nice way to say that my form completely stunk, and I had a long way to go before I could pass the test.

The next day, he had me standing in the turtle posture (imagine a downhill skier in a tuck position, knees bent to ninety degrees, elbows in, and head down) for five minutes at a time. He then would push me on the shoulders and hips to make sure my structure was intact. I had suffered through double days in soccer, but this was even more grueling. This training pushed me past the limits of what I thought was possible. He often showed skepticism about how a white kid from California could master these internal martial arts. But I was not going to give up. I did the exercises another thousand times and then another thousand.

Six months later, I thought I was ready for the Tai Chi test with Master Chia. I found Master Chia and asked if he would test me in the form again. He smiled, as if to say, didn't we just do this? I started my form with much more confidence. Master Chia came around and pushed me a few times. I felt completely different from the last time I tested, more rooted and grounded. I moved through his pushes with greater ease and effortlessness. He chuckled, as if to say, now let's see what you can really do. He demanded that I perform the advanced movements, and as I did, he began to lean on my back and yank on my arms. At first, I wanted to confront his force with force, but I remembered what I had learned from the tai chi classics: "Don't push the river, let the energy move through you." I relaxed and channeled his force into my center. I expanded my energy and pushed him backward. He grinned casually and nodded. "Good," he said. I had passed.

During my trips to Thailand, I would also venture off to other countries in Asia to study with other masters. I studied bodywork and pressure points in China and Japan. Over the years, I completed two-week silent retreats with nine hours of meditation a day. I meditated for ten days in complete darkness. I trained with tai chi masters in Hong Kong and Indonesia.

Back in the United States, I spent four years studying Chinese medicine and became a licensed Chinese medical doctor and acupuncturist. I wanted to understand the ancient theories and practices that had allowed for such a profound understanding of the human body, mind, and soul. At the time, I was on staff with Deepak Chopra and facilitated some of his workshops on MindBody Medicine. I completed numerous yoga intensives, stood on my head, and could almost get my ankles behind my ears (soccer players have tight hips). I wanted to absorb everything from as many different teachers and disciplines as I could to understand where their teachings merged and validated the insights into life that I was learning.

What I finally realized was that these practices and the Eastern approach to health that I was learning were not about extremes or competition; it wasn't about who could stretch the farthest or whose tai chi form was the best. It was all about an inner awareness and an awakening of inner potential. All of these teachers and traditions had many similarities, but the most important was to maintain balance. One of my teachers told me, "To maintain a garden all you need to do is give it a little water and sunlight each day." He explained that my practice should be the same—a little bit every day. That is what I hope to offer you in this book. A little bit of the essential elements—every day.

The book is a culmination of my studies through Asia, my personal daily practice, and what I've learned after teaching thousands of people these skills. What I have realized is that you don't have to spend years in a monastery or hiding out in a cave to get enormous benefits from tai chi, Zen, or yoga. In fact, all you need is 7 Minutes in the Morning or 7 Minutes in the Evening to transform your life. Think of this 7-minute workout as a distillation of the most complete full-body, energizing routines from the four-thousand-year-old traditions of tai chi, qi gong, and yoga combined with research on Western fitness and strength training.

Don't take my word for it—try it yourself for one month, and experience the difference.

2

East Meets West:
Your Body, Mind, and Spirit

Throughout my travels and training I have met some amazing people who seemed to glow with an inner radiance. To me these people were ageless, healthy, and full of vitality. I wanted to know their secrets. The knowledge and experience that I discovered during my travels was beyond Western medicine and transcended Western fitness routines. To really see the magic, I had to both understand my Western upbringing and see beyond it.

In the West we are typically trained to specialize, to segregate, and to compartmentalize. For example, if you have a physical injury, you see a doctor. If you have mental or emotional challenges, you visit a psychologist. If you have spiritual concerns, you seek the advice of a pastor, priest, or rabbi. This is how it has worked in our culture since the rise of modern medicine. There is great benefit from this system and it allows for great improvements in many specific areas.

The downfall of this paradigm is that we become fragmented. In reality, we are not segregated into the body, mind, and spirit. Putting up a fence between you and your neighbor doesn't mean that the earth is divided underneath.

From the Eastern perspective the body, mind, and spirit are a continuum, and the integrative whole is more important than the separate parts. Take water, for example. It can be in three different states—solid (ice), liquid (water), or gas (steam). Yet in each of these states, at the fundamental level, it is still H_2O. The same applies for us: The physical body is the densest form of energy, like ice; the mind and the emotions are more liquid, like water; and the spirit is like mist, more effervescent. One reason why people are so unhappy and unsatisfied, according to Eastern medicine, is that they feel disconnected, disjointed, and out of touch with this feeling of wholeness.

Eastern medicine describes how each of these elements— body, mind, and spirit—influence one another. For example, negative emotional energy and stress have a negative influence on the health of the body. Poor health, on the other hand, will have a negative influence on emotions and mind. The relationship is reciprocal. Imagine that you are in a beautiful place, like Hawaii—white sand beaches, perfect weather, crystal-clear water. Now imagine that you have the stomach flu. An unhealthy state in the body will limit your experience of joy. The energy of the body, mind, and spirit is part of one continual cycle.

We are more than all of our separate parts; more than organs, tissue, and muscles; more than emotions, thoughts, and feelings; more than our religious beliefs and cultural ideologies. We are the unity of all of these seemingly separate facets.

There are many different ways to accomplish our goals. Both Eastern and Western medicine have accomplished great feats in treating diseases, saving lives, and improving the quality of life. The East and West achieve this through completely different styles, each shaped by a unique paradigm.

As it stands now, our Western health-care model revolves around pain and sickness. If no one gets sick, no one gets paid. Conventional medicine differs from holistic medicine in that it is passive rather than dynamically proactive. Doctors give you things to take and procedures to do. Holistic medicine focuses on prevention and determining the root cause of a problem, not just its symptoms.

In Asia, there were and still are places where the health-care model is reversed. Clients pay their health-care practitioner a monthly fee as long as they stay healthy; when they get sick, they stop paying. Imagine a system where your health-care practitioner is this motivated to continually keep you healthy. It is a complete paradigm shift. How different would our Western medical system be if this were the practice today? As the saying goes, *What you put your attention on grows.*

When a health-care model focuses on prevention and wellness, these qualities flourish, like the sports coach telling his players that a good offense creates a good defense. By being proactive and focusing on health, we become stronger and more resilient, and even when we do get sick, it is often for a much shorter period of time.

True healing goes to the source of the problem and uproots the pattern of disease. Focusing only on symptoms is like trying to hold Ping-Pong balls under water—they eventually spring back up in many different directions. In the same way, masking symptoms often creates other health issues. For example, taking anti-inflamatory medications for an extended period of time sometimes can cause life-threatening damage to the internal organs. Real healing solutions lie in our ability to prevent problems before they arise or to seek long-term solutions in a holistic manner.

Pharmaceutical drugs temporarily alleviate pain, diminish anxiety and depression, or kill hostile germs in the body. Yet the root causes of our ailments are often left untouched. The containment, suppression, or elimination of symptomatic problems does not sustain vitality or vibrant health. Pharmaceutical treatment of secondary symptoms prunes the branches of our health problems while ignoring the roots. And these short-term solutions often come with long-term costs.

Despite continual advances in medical technology, we have more illness and pain than ever before. This is not to say that Western medicine is not truly amazing. It is. Just look at all the medical wonders it has achieved. Nothing compares to Western medicine when it comes to emergencies, vaccines, or finding solutions to life-threatening diseases. But this approach falls short when it comes to creating abundant energy, intrinsic health, and a sense of integration within. The East reminds us to focus on enhancing our life force energy and becoming healthy from the inside out.

As Western medicine takes an increasingly holistic approach to health, the practice becomes more aligned with the philosophy of Eastern medicine. Western medicine is starting to recognize how stress and negative emotions can cause all kinds of problems in the body. Prevention begins with stress management and alleviating excess mental and physical tension.

There is a saying in Chinese medicine: *Trying to get healthy after you are sick is like digging a well when you are dying of thirst.* The idea here is to focus on your health while you are healthy. This is not to say that if you are sick or in pain there is nothing to do. It just means that wherever you are on your path to health and vitality, now is the best time to begin.

From an Eastern perspective, and more and more a Western medical perspective, prevention is the key to lasting health and happiness. In taking charge of your own preventive health, I am not suggesting that you start performing acupuncture on yourself or that you start concocting herbal potions. Let the professionals do what they do best. But controlling your own health destiny is possible. By doing a little energy cultivation and stress clearing each day, your entire system will become much more resilient and strong. That is what *7 Minutes of Magic* is all about—a little bit of water and sunshine every day.

Think of this book as a guide for prevention, a simple way to have your well dug and the water of health and vitality flowing. The 7 Minutes of Magic program is a quick and easy way to prevent low energy, stress, and premature aging. The routines will keep you feeling, looking, and staying younger than your calendar age.

Stress

Stress is a buzzword. It shows up everywhere—magazines, newspapers, doctors' offices, at work, and on TV. You probably can't make it through a single day without seeing or hearing the word.

In our modern world, life has become ever more fast-paced and is increasingly complex and, in a word, stressful. Even with our advances in technology, our bodies are still the same. Lights turn night into day, stores make it easy to get whatever we want at any time, yet our bodies still operate on the same cycles and rhythms as they have for thousands of years. It's no wonder that balance is so difficult to achieve when we push ourselves in so many unnatural ways.

This type of lifestyle leaves us too depleted to get sufficient exercise, relaxation, or play, or even to spend quality time with our families. This energy-depleting way of life and chronic stress lead to anxiety, fatigue, depression, a weakened immune system, and a host of serious physical and psychological ailments.

These problems arise not only from stress itself, but in the way we handle stress. The steady rise of drug use, addictions, unhealthy relationships, zoning out with entertainment (too much TV), excessive shopping, and purchasing of material possessions are all examples of how we respond to stress in detrimental ways. This is especially true if we feel a lack of support or a lack of inner resources.

It isn't always possible to remove an outer problem. You can't always quit your job, make your child behave, get out of a traffic jam, or heal a serious injury. But you can change your response and your inner state of consciousness. Dealing effectively with the stresses and problems in your life is a choice. When you have more energy and vitality, problems and stress don't seem so overwhelming. By taking time for yourself, you will cultivate the energy you need to handle your problems more skillfully and effectively.

The stress response evolved for a good reason—to protect you from danger. I became all too familiar with this response early in my life. On my thirteenth birthday, my father took me to Alaska, a sort of initiation into manhood, an adventure into the wild. On our second day in the bush, we were hiking along a beautiful trail next to a river, watching the salmon jump up a waterfall. As we stopped to admire the spectacular scenery, a huge grizzly came out of the trees and onto the trail a mere four feet from us. His head was bigger than my entire body. I froze. My mouth went dry and my heart felt as if it were going to pop out of my chest.

At that moment, all these bodily changes were basically giving me a choice—I could put up my dukes and have a wrestling match with the bear, or I could find the quickest way to escape. Scientifically, this is known as the fight-or-flight response.

I had heard the fishermen and the local Alaskan folks say not to run if you came face to face with a bear, but at that moment, my mind went blank and my legs moved like a roadrunner. Both my dad and I were sprinting away down the trail and scrambling up into a tree faster than a squirrel. Of course the bear was much more interested in the salmon, but we still stayed in that tree until the bear walked off and looked for lunch elsewhere.

Physiologically, here's what happened to my body in that situation: My sympathetic nervous system kicked in to high gear. The hypothalamus (a gland in the brain) activated the pituitary, which released a hormone called ACTH (adrenocorticotropic hormone) into the bloodstream. This hormone went to my adrenal glands, which in turn produced more adrenaline (also known as epinephrine) along with other hormones called glucocorticoids (cortisol is an example). This set off an array of biochemical changes in my body:

- My heart rate sped up, and my blood pressure went up (more blood was pumped to the muscles and lungs).

- My breath was rapid, nostrils flaring, causing an increased supply of air to my lungs.

- Blood was directed away from my skin and internal organs and was sent to my brain and skeletal muscles. My muscles tensed.

I felt stronger (although not strong enough to wrestle the bear!).

- My blood would clot faster, just in case the bear actually caught me and tossed me around like in a World Wrestling Federation match. This would repair damage done to the arteries much faster.

- My pupils dilated, giving me better vision (not so necessary when a one-thousand-pound grizzly is four feet away—I could see him very clearly).

- My liver converted glycogen into glucose, which teamed up with free fatty acids to supply me with fuel and quick energy.

Under these circumstances, the fight-or-flight response was totally appropriate. This same bodily reaction served the caveman when confronted with a saber-toothed tiger. Yet, as a modern man, this same response can be elicited while sitting in a traffic jam or giving a presentation to a group of colleagues. In fact, any perceived stress can put a person into this fight-or-flight state.

This incredibly important, life-preserving stress reaction is hardwired into our system. But the reality is, in our modern society, we are required to deal with very few grizzly bears or life-threatening stresses. The problem is that our bodies do not know the difference between a grizzly and a traffic jam, so we react in a similar way.

In the situation of the grizzly bear, this stress response has an outlet. The body uses the energy to get away or fight off the enemy. In a traffic jam, the stress response has no outlet and runs around the body like a caged tiger. Over time, this type of stress is detrimental to our health.

In today's modern jungle, public speaking, a disgruntled spouse, dealing with a difficult client, having a demanding deadline, and raising children are all stressful, but not life-threatening. When your body overreacts to stressful situations, the same stress hormones are released into the body as if you were in imminent danger. When this fight-or-flight response is repeatedly triggered, it wears down the body and mind. The stress response was designed to work best in short-term situations—not for the prolonged stress that we deal with on a routine basis.

Every bodily system is affected by stress. The statistics are striking: 112 million people in the U.S. take some form of medication for stress-related symptoms. One reason this number is so high is that stress seeps into all aspects of our lives, both physically and psychologically, and it can exacerbate previous health-related symptoms.

From muscle tension to headaches, from irritable bowel syndrome to acid indigestion, from heart disease to cancer, the steady rise in stress-related illness reflects our inability to cope with our lifestyles. This gives birth to a billion-dollar health-care industry that at times masks the deeper problems of the roots of stress. The numerous medical studies on Eastern practices, like qi gong, yoga, tai chi, and meditation, have shown that they reverse the effects of many stress-related ailments.

Among the signs and symptoms of stress on the body are:

- Tight muscles and body aches

- Fatigue, lethargy

- Shallow, short breathing

- Chest tightness, rapid pulse

- Heartburn, indigestion, diarrhea, constipation

- Dry mouth and throat

- Excessive sweating, clammy hands, cold hands or feet

- Skin irritations, eczema

- Nail biting, fidgeting, hair twirling

- Lowered libido

- Overeating or loss of appetite

- Insomnia, excessive dreaming

- Increased use of alcohol and drugs

Among the psychological signs of stress are:

- Frustration, irritability, anger

- Impatience

- Worry and anxiety

- Sadness, depression

- Insecurity, fear

- Panic attacks

- Moodiness, emotional instability

- Intrusive and racing thoughts

- Memory lapses, difficulty concentrating

- Indecision

- Loss of a sense of humor

Stress robs people of many of life's pleasures and deprives them of many of life's satisfactions—including laughter. Stress can take many forms—work pressure, financial concerns, health issues, relationship challenges, being single, having a baby, taking on a mortgage, or having too little time for oneself.

The following indicate some of the problems many of us in the United States face:

- **Stress and Daily Life:** According to the American Medical Association, 89 percent of adults describe experiencing high levels of stress.

- **Stress and Medical Visits:** According to the American Institute of Stress, 75 to 90 percent of adult visits to primary care physicians are for stress-related problems.

- **Stress and Work:** According to a study by the George Pfeiffer WorkCare Group, one million employees are absent on an average workday because of stress-related problems.

- **Stress Can Be Deadly:** More people have heart attacks on Monday morning at nine a.m. than at any other time of the week.

- **Stress Can Cause Illness:** Stress is linked to the following—hypertension, heart attack, diabetes, asthma, chronic pain, allergies, headache, backache, skin disorders, cancer, immune system weakness, and a decrease in white blood cell count.

- **Stress and Sex:** Stress can affect sexual performance and rob you of your libido. Disturbed sexual performance may appear in the form of premature ejaculation, erectile dysfunction, and other forms of difficulty in reaching orgasm.

- **Stress and Cholesterol:** Stress is more powerful than diet in influencing cholesterol levels. Several studies, including one of medical students around exam time and another of accountants during tax season, have shown significant increases in cholesterol levels during stressful times, when there was little change in diet.

- **Stress and Heart Disease:** Stress is now considered a major risk factor in heart disease, right up there with smoking, being overweight, and lack of exercise.

- **Stress and Digestion:** Stress can affect the secretion of acid in your stomach and can speed up or slow down the process of peristalsis. Constipation, diarrhea, gas, bloating, irritable bowel syndrome, and weight gain can be stress related.

- **Stress and Muscle Tension:** Your muscles are prime targets for stress. Under stress, your muscles contract and tense. This muscle tension affects the nerves, blood vessels, organs, skin, and bones. Chronically tenses muscles can result in a variety of conditions and disorders, including muscle spasms, pain, and teeth grinding.

- **Stress and the Immune System:** Stress hampers the immune system, and stressful life events can bring about colds, flus, and allergies.

- **Stress and Risk of Stroke:** Severe stress is one of the most potent risk factors for stroke—more so than high blood pressure—even fifty years after the initial stress-inducing trauma. In a study conducted by Dr. Lawrence Brass at the Yale Medical School, of 556 veterans of World War II, the rate of stroke among those who had been prisoners of war was eight times higher than among those not captured.

Regardless of whether you are working from an Eastern or Western approach, there is a fundamental question that health practitioners have puzzled over for years: Why does one person catch a virus while someone else does not? Increasingly the evidence is leading us to look at energy levels, vitality, and response to stress. One such study, by Dr. Sheldon Cohen at Carnegie Mellon University, took four hundred people and intentionally exposed them to the common-cold viruses. Those who had the most stressful life events were more than twice as likely to develop colds after exposure as people who had the fewest.

Researchers have now coined a term for the study of how stress and low energy affect the immune system. It is called psychoneuroimmunology (try to say *that* seven times fast). In short, stress can compromise your immune system, rendering it less effective in resisting bacteria and viruses.

The good news is that stress can be alleviated with the right exercises, movements, stretches, and relaxation techniques. This is exactly what the 7 Minutes of Magic program is designed to do. It's about tapping into your resources so that the inevitable stress and tensions of life make you more productive instead of self-destructive. These seven-minute sequences give you the ability to transform stress into a catalyst for creativity and manifesting what you want out of life.

Energy

Energy is that elusive quality we are all seeking. It is that vital force that makes life exciting, fun, creative, and joyful.

Call it *qi* (Chinese), *prana* (Indian), *ruach* (Hebrew), spirit, youthfulness, or vibrant health, energy is what we crave. Quantum physicists describe energy as the nature of the universe but can't really explain what it actually is. You can allude to it, you can feel it and perceive it, but it is beyond our best mental concepts and explanations. Instinctively we know that the more energy we have, the better we feel.

Energy is the invisible, immaterial substance that propagates life and animates our bodies with movement. It gives birth to our thoughts, emotions, and consciousness. Energy describes and is infused in both the infinite space of the universe and the infinitesimal space of the smallest particles. It is the spiral dance of the planets, the magnetism between the electron and proton, and the attraction between male and female. Energy is in the air we breathe, the food we eat, and the emotions we feel. It is the force that allows the planets, stars, and galaxies to work in perfect harmony. Mountains arising, forests growing, rivers flowing, and all life proliferating are expressions of this life force.

Quantum physicists and mystics from all ages agree that we are literally made of and are living within a limitless sea of energy. How is it then, that we suffer from chronic low energy, fatigue, and poor health? Medical surveys show that lack of energy and high levels of stress are the biggest complaints in physicians' offices today.

Think about it this way: If the power lines go down or flicker on and off during a storm, everything in the house stops working or only works sporadically. Without electricity, we have no heat, we can't cook our food, watch TV, or use the computer. If we apply the same principle to our minds and bodies, we see that low energy causes shortages in our overall vitality, our stress levels, our libido, our creativity, and our enjoyment of life, and in the way we metabolize food.

The choices we make every day, from exercise to diet, change the way we feel and work from the inside out. As we cultivate more energy within ourselves, the stresses that we normally face aren't so overwhelming. As our energy increases, so does our ability to handle stress and create effective solutions. It's when we are depleted that stress seeps into our bodies and minds.

In Eastern terms, the more energy we have circulating in the body, the healthier we are. Abundant energy manifests in the body as better functioning organs, more flexibility in the muscles, supple joints, and balanced emotions. Loss of internal energy creates fatigue, tension, low metabolism, inability to cope with stress, insomnia, depression, and turbulent thoughts.

Energy level is a great indicator of our general health. A Yale University study found that energy levels had the highest correlation with general-health status and were the best predictors of both physical and psychological health over time. Energetic people, the study showed, are generally healthy, whereas the enervated are often ill, becoming ill, fighting off illness, or struggling with their low-energy condition. Illness, apathy, fatigue, anxiety, chronic stress, depression, and the like are all signs that we are becoming depleted.

Cultivating More Energy

Nature pulses with energy. In the Eastern forms of exercise, tapping into the abundant energy all around us and within us is one of the goals. Sometimes cultivating more energy is as simple as getting out of our own way, of letting go of stress, tension, old emotions, and discordant thoughts. Abundant energy is not something that we have to create or make. It is always there, wanting to flow, wanting to express itself as creativity and balance.

Searching for energy in the material world, as we so often do, often leads to disappointment. It is important to remember that the path to more energy is not through acquiring things. What we want in the material world is a reflection of an inner feeling—security, fulfillment, health, power, excitement, youth, and vitality. These are all inner qualities. One of my teachers calls this incessant desire for material goods the search for "dragon eggs." In other words, it is a search for something that doesn't exist.

To cultivate energy from the inside is something that lasts—a way to go to the source of energy and allow it to grow. Happiness and joy already exist inside you. The notion that acquiring material possessions will elicit this inner quality only leads to continual grasping of external things. Going outside of ourselves in a quest for happiness it is like trying to capture waves by scooping up the ocean in a bucket. By cultivating energy from within, you can enjoy the material world without attachment. The material world is for our enjoyment and experience, but when we approach it from internal balance and strength, we can appreciate our possessions without being controlled by them.

The key to happiness and vitality is balance: harmony in your life in every area, both internal and external, including diet, exercise, work, relationships, sleep, play, and contemplation.

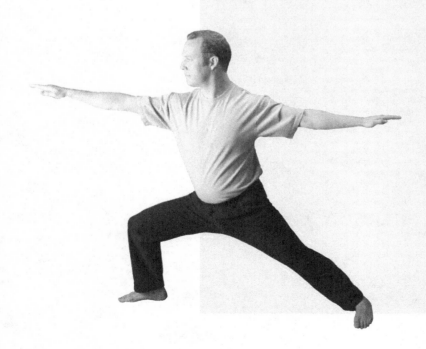

PART II

The Flows

Think of a river moving down a mountain—effortless, liquid, powerful. The morning and evening routines mirror the movements of nature and the natural rhythms of the body to build energy and vitality. There is no lack of energy in nature, only cycles and rhythms. These flows are designed to get you connected to your inner cycles and rhythms.

The morning routine wakes the body up as nature comes to life, so you can charge your body with the energy of life itself. The evening routine clears stress and tension, calms the mind, and prepares the body for deep, restful sleep.

The routines themselves are continuous, each movement giving rise to the next in one cohesive flow. No movement is wasted, giving you the most benefit in the least amount of time and with the least effort. Tai chi and qi gong are called "the art of effortless power" because of their simplicity and rhythm, one movement giving rise to the next. Here, each posture and each stretch combine together in a flow to give maximum benefit.

Stretching is important to the body because it clears residual tension as it builds up in the muscles. When the muscles get tight and tense, circulation is impeded, creating stagnation in the body's energy system. Anything in nature that is full of youthful life force is supple. A tree that is healthy is resilient; if you bend a branch down, it springs back. If the tree is old or stiff, when you pull it, the branch will break. This same idea applies to our bodies; if we want to cultivate youthful vitality, becoming supple and flexible is a necessity. As the Taoist sage Lao Tzu says in the *Tao Te Ching,* "Those that are supple are disciples of life. Those that are brittle are disciples of death."

Health is an ongoing process, not a goal that is ever reached. It is a daily journey; you are either taking steps toward health or away from it every day. That is the beauty of this program; you only need seven minutes a day to increase your energy, vitality, and overall health. I hope that after these flowing exercise routines have become a part of your life you, too, will use the word *magic* to describe the changes that you experience in your body and mind.

3

7 Minutes of Magic in the Morning

The morning routine begins with the Core Flow, focusing on the lower back and abdominal area. This area is the center of the body, the storehouse where energy and vitality originate. By opening this area, the lower back becomes flexible and supple, the abs become strong and supportive, and the hips become open and balanced. The core of the body is called the Tan Tien in tai chi and qi gong. Tan Tien means "reservoir," a powerhouse to store and tap into the body's innate vitality.

From the core, the sequence continues with the Upper Body Flow, focusing on strength through the shoulders and chest, and flexibility through the back. Combining elements of yoga and upper-body conditioning, we are able to stretch and release tension as well as strengthen to create stronger muscles and burn fat.

Next in the series is the Lower Body Flow, focusing on stretching the hamstrings, opening the hips, and strengthening all the muscles in the legs and buttocks. This sequence includes lunges and squats to fire up the body's metabolism by engaging the biggest muscles in the body and building power in the legs.

Your body can burn fat more efficiently if you build up large muscle groups like your core, chest, quadriceps, hamstrings, and gluteal muscles. Focus on these and you will work more muscle fibers than if you targeted smaller ones, and you will add lean muscle to your frame. The more muscle fibers you utilize, the more lean muscle tissue you'll develop, which really boosts your metabolism.

The Full Body Flow follows as a way to stretch all the major muscles in the body. This series of movements will help alleviate tightness and tension throughout the entire body. It also creates balance between the front (the abs, hips, chest, and quadriceps) and the back (the spine, muscles of the back, buttocks, and hamstrings). This allows the body to find equilibrium with no muscular tension.

The routine continues with the Energy Flow, bringing in elements of tai chi and qi gong and pressure points to awaken key energy lines. This sequence awakens the dormant energy within the body and allows it to circulate. Elements of this flow come from the martial arts side of tai chi and help develop internal power and abundant vitality.

After the internal energy is awakened, it is circulated in the body with the Breath Flow, which helps to bring more oxygen into the lungs through deep breathing. The increased intake of oxygen carries energy to every cell, creating health and wellness from the inside out. Deeper breathing helps athletes perform better, creates clarity in the mind, and releases emotional stress.

The sequence ends with the Mind Flow, a way to focus your intention and plant seeds for how you want your day to unfold. By visualizing and focusing attention on the rest of the day, you are tapping into the power of your mind. Your creative power, like anything else, is strengthened when it is used. By focusing it every day we become cocreators in the flow of our lives, manifesting what's in our hearts and minds with less effort.

As with all exercise routines, make sure each of the flows feels good for your body. If any one of the exercises doesn't feel good, try some of the modifications or skip it and spend a little more time on the other flows.

Core Flow

This routine begins from the center—your core—and is designed to strengthen the abdomen, hips, and lower back. It also creates a greater range of motion in the lower back and hips, bringing in the principles of yoga, qi gong, and Pilates to energize your center.

1. Lie on your back. Hug your knees to the chest.

This is one of the simplest exercises to perform. You see it in yoga, qi gong, and even physical therapy. Why? Because it starts to open the lumbar spine, the core of the back. It is a good stretch for releasing tension and pain in the lower back and prevents back pain from occurring in the future. Countless people wake up with lower back pain. This posture eases the back into opening and clearing stiffness.

Take 1 deep breath.

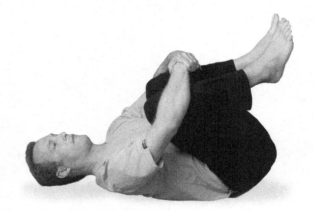

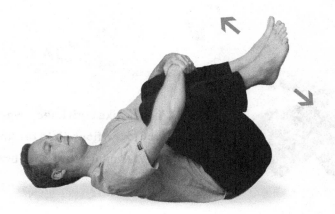

**2. Now try rocking a little bit from the right to the left.
Do this 7 times to each side.**

Notice how the rocking massages the lower back into the floor. The kidneys and adrenal glands are located in this area of the back, just above the last rib where it's attached to the spine. In our society we are constantly stimulating the adrenals with coffee, smoking, and entertainment. We get addicted to the adrenaline rush, to the fight-or-flight response. This can wreak havoc on the body. By massaging the back into the floor, you give a natural stimulation to the adrenal glands. This is a great way to wake the body up without caffeine, from the inside out. You do not have to stop drinking coffee, but it can become a choice rather than a necessity for making it through the day.

3. Twist. Take both knees over to the right side, all the way to the floor. Hold the knees down with the right hand and turn the upper body and head to the left.

Hold for 7 seconds.

4. Do the twist to the other side. Take both knees over to the left side, all the way to the floor. Hold the knees down with the left hand and turn the upper body and head to the right.

Hold for 7 seconds.

Again, this is a classic stretch to open the lower back, stretch the rib cage, and bring the breath deeper into the lungs. Deep breathing is the secret to getting more out of this stretch. See if you can bring your breath down through the ribs and feel the expansion in your lower back and abdomen. Twisting is a great way to create suppleness in your spine. After our teenage years, the only way to increase the flow of spinal fluid in the joints is to do the appropriate stretching. This is one of the best stretches—sometimes you can literally feel the disks between the joints filling up with that nutritive spinal fluid.

More Magic for the Back

Bridge. Bring both feet flat onto the floor with your knees bent. On an inhale, slowly raise your hips upward toward the ceiling, bringing your back off the floor. Lift all the way up onto your shoulders, squeezing the muscles in your buttocks as you come up. Then slowly roll down on an exhale, feeling each vertebra making contact with the floor. Do this sequence 7 times.

The bridge is an excellent exercise to strengthen the lower back, open the hips, and increase range of motion in the spine. It also brings energy into the central nervous system.

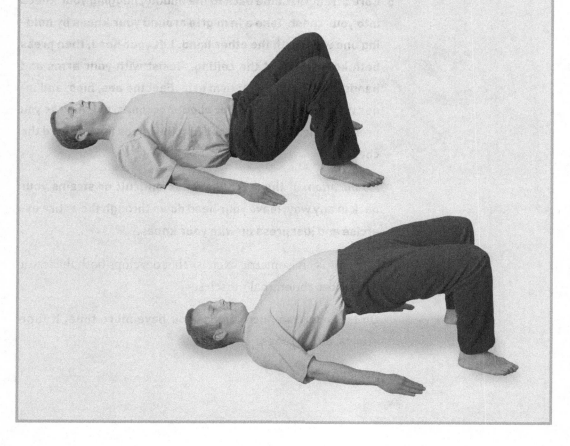

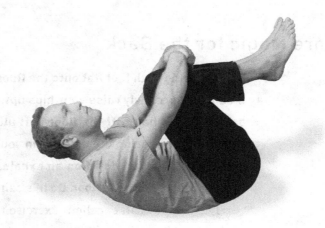

5. **Core Strength. Come back to the middle, hugging your knees into your chest. Take a firm grip around your knees by holding one wrist with the other hand. Lift your head, then press both knees toward the ceiling. Resist with your arms and hands, maintaining that firm grip. Feel the abs, hips, and inner thighs working. Hold for about 7 seconds, exhaling as you press. Inhale as you relax and hug the knees back toward the chest.**

Modification: **If this exercise is too difficult or strains your neck in any way, leave your head down through the entire exercise and just press up with your knees.**

This is an isometric exercise that develops both the lower and upper abdominal muscles.

Do this exercise once, unless you have more time. If time allows, do it 3 times.

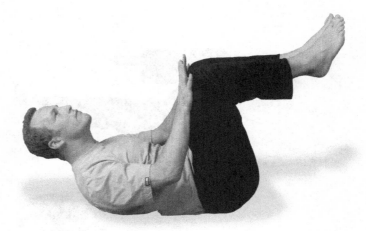

6. **Next, place your hands on top of your thighs, just below your knees. Lift your head and press your knees toward your face, resisting with your hands. Hold for about 7 seconds, exhaling as you press. Then hug your knees into your chest.**

   This exercise works the lower abs and the psoas muscle (the muscle that supports your lower spine and hips, pronounced *soaz*). Your body might vibrate slightly—this is how you know your core muscles are really working.

   Modification: **If this exercise is too difficult or strains your neck in any way, leave the head down through the entire exercise and just press your knees toward your face.**

7. **Bring your feet flat onto the floor and interlock your fingers behind your head. Bring your left elbow to your right knee, then your right elbow to your left knee. Go back and forth like this at an even pace for about 14 seconds. Breathe evenly and naturally through the entire exercise.**

   This bicycle-type movement works the entire abdominal area. Studies show that this particular exercise works the core of the body better than any other exercise. The rotating

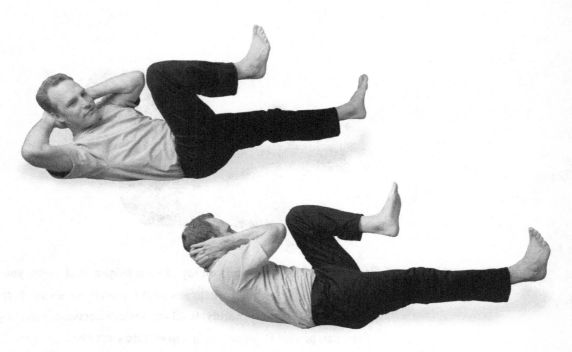

movement engages the spinal muscles and internal and external obliques, the supportive muscles along the sides of the abdomen.

Modification: **If this exercise is too difficult or strains your neck in any way, leave your head down through the entire exercise and just bicycle your legs.**

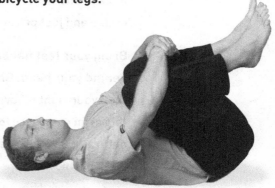

8. Hug your knees to your chest.

More Magic for the Core: Pull the Bow

Straighten both legs with your hands at your sides. Slowly lift your legs 6 inches off the floor with your feet flexed. At the same time, lift your upper body off the floor and extend your hands toward your feet. Exhale and hold for 7 seconds.

This exercise strengthens the lower abdomen, which is part of your body's core. The core is made up of the abdominal muscles themselves, as well as the obliques and the psoas muscle. The psoas muscle is particularly important because of its relation to the lower back. Sometimes called "the seat of the soul," this muscle is crucial in supporting the structure of the body. The psoas attaches to the lumbar spine and runs along the back of the abdomen into the hip. Back trouble often comes from a weak psoas muscle.

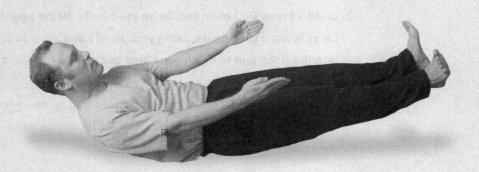

Upper Body Flow

The Upper Body Flow delivers strength and power to your shoulders, arms, and upper back. It also develops flexibility and suppleness through the spine. The spine is the source of power and energy for the entire body. Having a strong upper body is nothing without the foundation of a strong and open spine. This flow has elements of the Sun Salutation from yoga and conditioning exercises for the chest, shoulders, lats, and upper back.

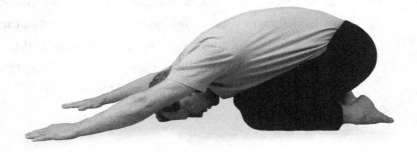

1. **Child's Pose. Roll over and lie on your belly. Bring your buttocks toward your heels, using your hands and arms to press into the floor and to bring your hips back. Hold for one deep breath.**

    Child's Pose is a rejuvenating posture that helps to gently stimulate the central nervous system, while easing tension in the spine.

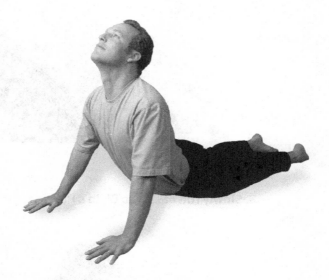

2. **Cobra. Slowly slide your hands forward. Allow your upper body to follow, keeping your chest close to the floor. When your chest and shoulders are between your hands, lightly press up into Cobra Pose. Feel the opening through your shoulders and upper back, enlivening your entire spine. Take one deep breath.**

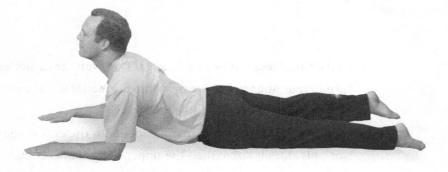

Modification: **If you have back pain or the full pose feels too difficult, you can come up on your elbows instead of pressing all the way up on your hands. Remember, make sure all the exercises feel comfortable in your body.**

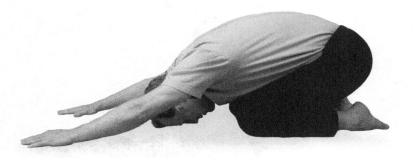

3. Slowly roll back into Child's Pose.

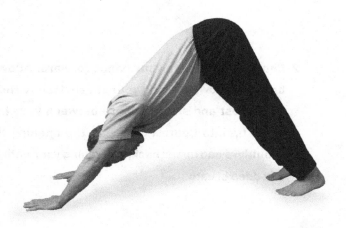

4. Mountain. Press up onto all fours. Curl your toes under, spread your fingers and press up into the Mountain, or as it is called in yoga, Downward-Facing Dog.

This posture delivers many benefits to the entire body. Not only does it strengthen the upper body, it also stretches the legs, elongates the back, and awakens the entire spine.

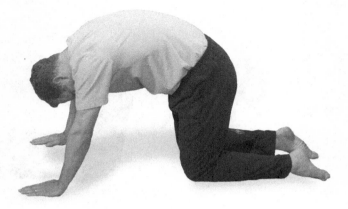

Modification: **Stay on all fours , round the back, and tuck your chin in toward the chest.**

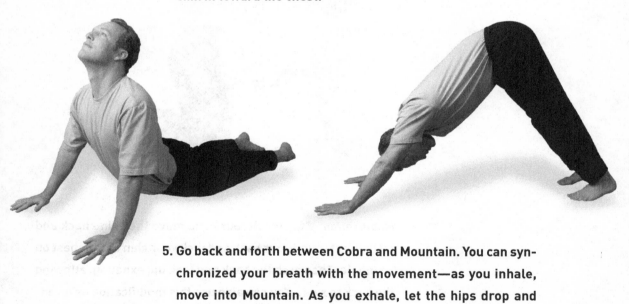

5. Go back and forth between Cobra and Mountain. You can synchronized your breath with the movement—as you inhale, move into Mountain. As you exhale, let the hips drop and press up into Cobra. Go back and forth 7 times.

This exercise is said to be one of the best exercises for a healthy spine and longevity.

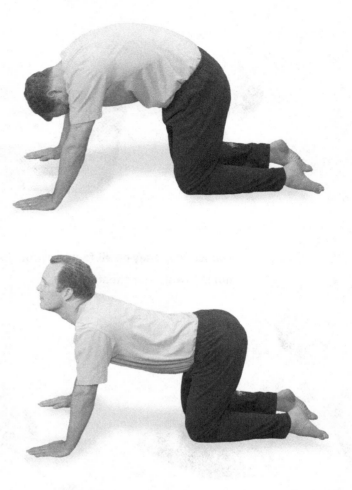

Modification: Stay on all fours and move the spine back and forth. First round your back and tuck your chin to the chest on an inhale. Then arch the back and look up, exhaling, allowing the back to sway. You can also use this modification as an additional exercise to stretch and relax the back.

More Magic for the Back

1. **Flying. Roll over onto your abdomen and extend both arms in front of you. Begin by lifting your head and right arm and left leg up off the floor. Hold for 7 seconds while exhaling.**

2. **Then, lift your left arm and your right leg up off the floor. Hold for another 7 seconds while exhaling.**

3. **Lift both arms and both legs off the floor at the same time. Hold for 7 seconds, again while exhaling.**

This exercise brings strength and energy into the lower back area. The lumbar area of the lower back is central to the entire body. A strong lower back maintains the structure and integrity of the entire body. This exercise also helps keep the tension in the lower back evenly distributed and facilitates proper alignment.

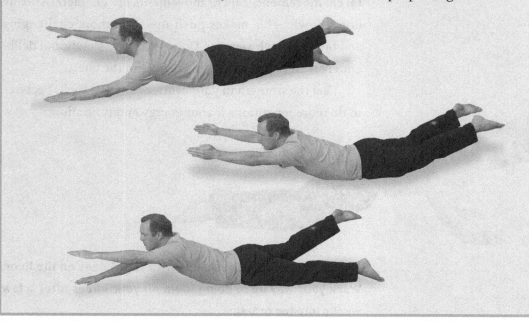

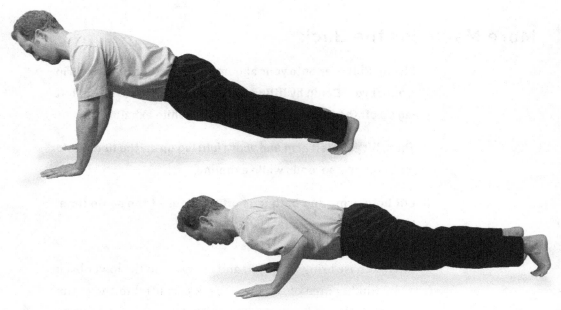

6. Tai Chi Push-Up. Finish this set with 7 slow push-ups. Lower down slowly and push up slowly, as if you were doing a slow tai chi movement. Tai chi movements are characteristically done slowly. This makes push-ups even more challenging and builds muscle quicker. Doing exercises slowly and deliberately better conditions the muscles in the chest.

Feel the strength in your arms, chest, and back. Feel free to do more repetitions if your energy and time allow.

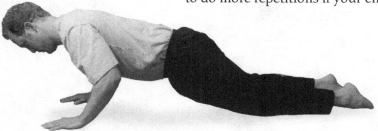

Modification: **Do the push-ups with your knees on the floor. Work your way up to doing them off your knees after a few weeks into the practice.**

Lower Body Flow

The lower body flow builds strength through the base of the body. As a tree is only as strong as its roots, so, too, do our bodies build strength from the legs upward. By working the legs and lower body, metabolism is increased, fat is burned, and our foundation becomes more solid.

1. **Forward Bend. From lying face down, step up, bringing your feet between your hands. Hinge forward at the waist and go into a forward bend. Hang forward from your waist with your knees slightly bent, arms dangling toward your feet.** Feel this posture stretching the hamstrings and opening your lower back. Take a moment to relax your neck and shoulders.

Take 2 deep breaths.

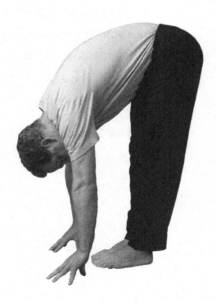

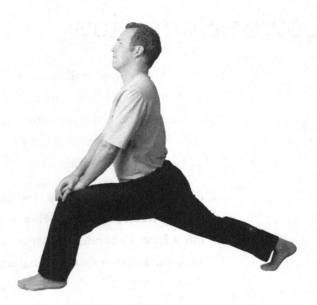

2. **Lunge. Bring your hands down to the floor by bending your knees. Step back with your right foot into a lunge, keeping your hands on the floor or, if it feels comfortable, bring them onto your front knee.** Feel the strength and power in your legs. This posture not only strengthens the legs but also opens the hips, creates support for the lower back, and stretches the hamstrings.

Hold for 7 seconds.

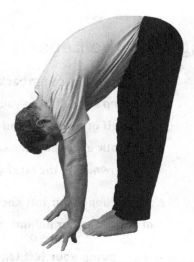

3. Step back up into a forward bend, with both feet together. Take one deep breath here.

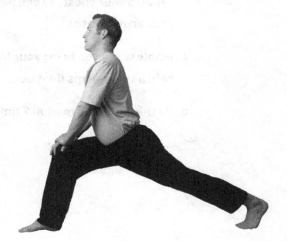

4. Again, bend your knees, bringing your hands down to the floor, then step back with your left leg, going into a lunge on the other side. Keep your hands on the floor or, if it feels comfortable, press both hands up to the front knee, stretching and strengthening.

Hold for 7 seconds.

More Magic for the Legs

1. **Lunge and Flow.** Step back with your right foot into a lunge. As you step back, flatten your right foot onto the floor, keeping yourself grounded. Bend your left knee and keep it directly over your ankle, making sure you can see your toes when you look down. Feel the strength and power in your left leg.

2. As you bend your left knee, float your arms out, one in front of you, the other behind you.

3. Next, pump your left leg slowly from being straight into a deep knee bend. As you straighten your left leg, your hands come to your chest. As you bend your left knee into the lunge, your arms float out.

4. Inhale when you bring your hands toward your chest, and exhale as your arms float out.

5. Do this pumping motion 7 times.

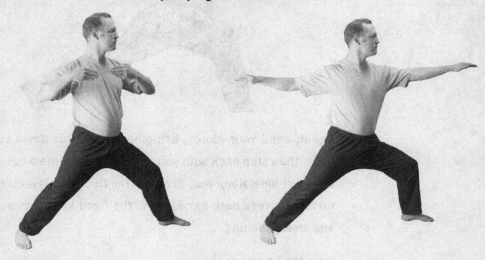

6. Step your right foot up next to your left foot. Hinge forward at your waist into a forward bend. Take one deep breath here.

7. Then step back with your left foot into a lunge. As you step back, flatten your left foot onto the floor. Bend your right knee, keeping it directly over your right ankle.

8. Pump your right leg, slowly letting your arms float out as you bend the knee. Then, bringing your arms and hands to your chest, straighten your leg.

9. Inhale as you bring your hands toward your chest, and exhale as you float your arms out.

10. Do this 7 times.

The lunge and pump creates both strength and flexibility in the legs, activating the large muscle groups. It is a powerful way to enhance your metabolism and create tone in the body.

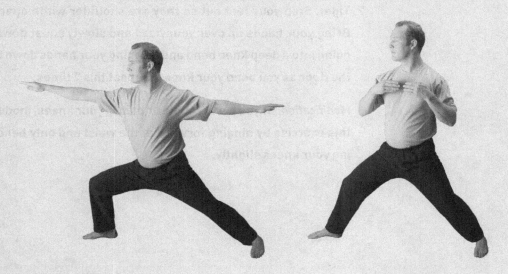

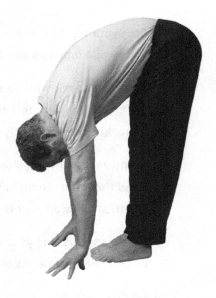

5. Again, step back up into a forward bend, with both feet together.

6. Slowly roll up to standing.

7. Tiger. Step your feet out so they are shoulder width apart. Bring your hands up over your head and slowly squat down, going into a deep knee bend and bringing your hands down to the floor as you bend your knees. Repeat this 7 times.

Modification: If you have trouble or pain in your knees, modify this exercise by hinging forward at the waist and only bending your knees slightly.

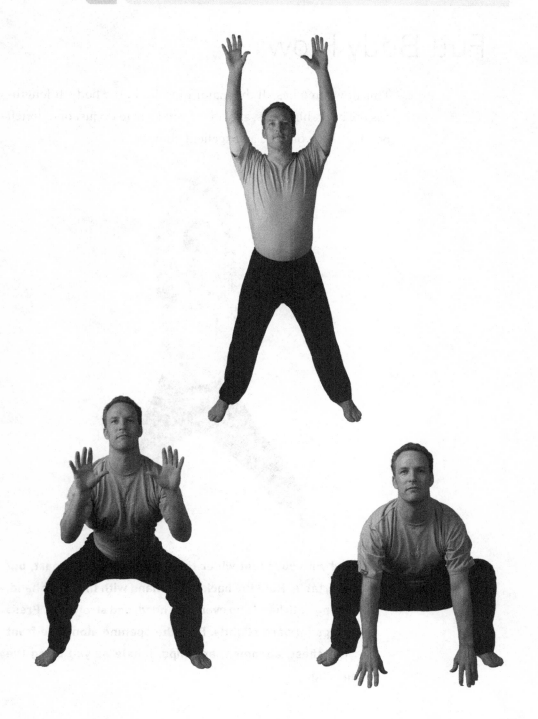

Full Body Flow

This flow stretches all the major muscles in the body. It length-ens the back, hips, legs, and abs. If you were to do just one stretch per day, this would be an excellent choice.

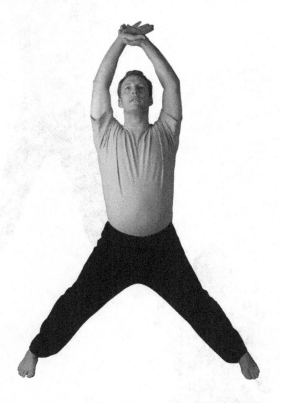

1. **Stand with your feet wider than shoulder width apart, but comfortable. Hold the back of one hand with the other hand, bringing both hands up over your head, and stretch up. Press the hips forward slightly. Feel the opening along the front of the chest, abdomen, and hips. Inhale as you bring the hands up.**

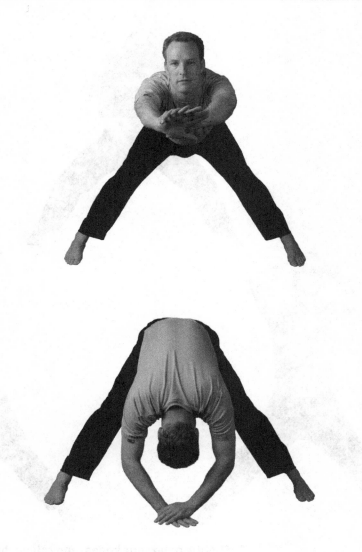

2. Extend your arms forward and stretch toward the floor. Exhale as you come down and feel the opening along the back of the legs.

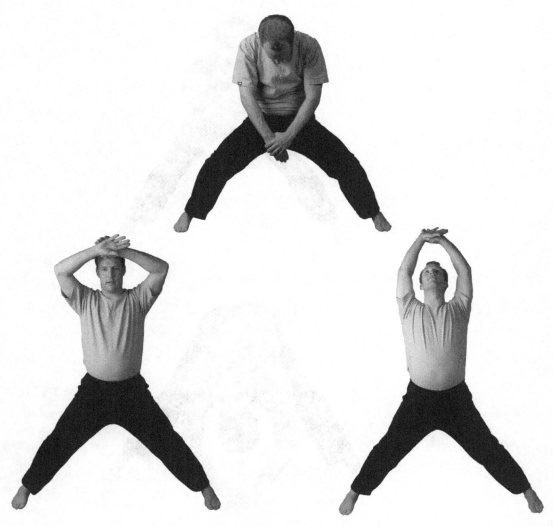

3. Slightly bend your knees, and roll up, bringing your hands up over your head. Press your hips forward, opening the front of the body. Inhale.

4. Again, extend out, going into a forward bend, stretching the back of the body and continuing this flowing stretch 7 times, reaching up and back as you inhale, then extending forward and down as you exhale.

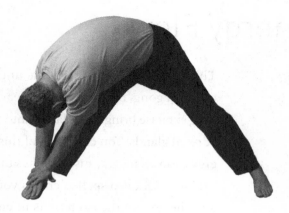

5. Keeping your feet apart, hang forward and stretch over to the right side, bringing your head toward your right knee. Take a deep breath.

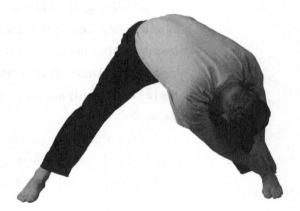

6. Repeat on the left side, bringing your head toward your left knee. Take a deep breath.

7. Come back to the center and roll up.

Energy Flow

This flow comes from the ancient exercise routine from China called qi gong, the exercises that gave birth to tai chi. The beginning exercise brings circulation into the lower back, kidneys, and adrenal glands. You can think of this sequence as an internal energy cappuccino because it wakes up the adrenal glands in a natural way. Qi (also spelled chi) is your life force or inner vitality, and the goal of the exercise is to cultivate high-quality energy. This is accomplished by stimulating vital pressure points and circulating the internal energy with a few basic movements.

1. **Knocking on the Door of Life. Bring your feet in, standing shoulder-width apart. Start a slow turning motion from the hips and waist, keeping the shoulders, arms, and upper back relaxed. Let the momentum from the center of your body (hips and waist) move your arms. As you continue, allow your arms to knock gently across your lower back and across your abdomen.**

   This stimulates a pressure point called the door of life, located directly behind the navel, on the spine. This point enhances overall vitality and energizes the central nervous system.

2. **Continue for 7 times in each direction.**

3. **Allow the movement to slowly unwind, and bring your arms back to your sides.**

4. **Breathe naturally and normally through the entire routine.**

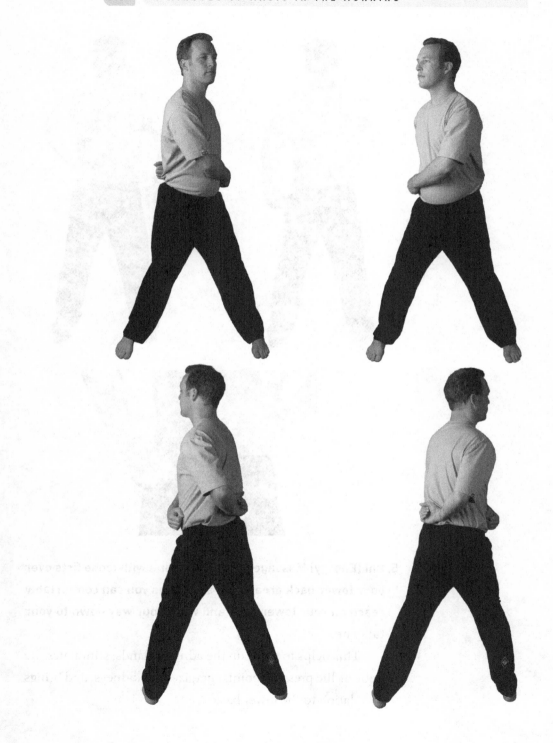

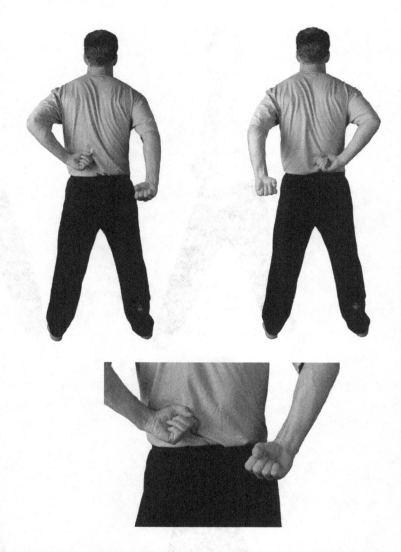

5. Chi (Energy) Massage. Start by tapping with loose fists over your lower back area. Start as high as you can comfortably reach on your lower back and work your way down to your tailbone.

This helps to wake up the adrenal glands, stimulates the door-of-life pressure point, energizes the kidneys, and brings circulation to the lower back.

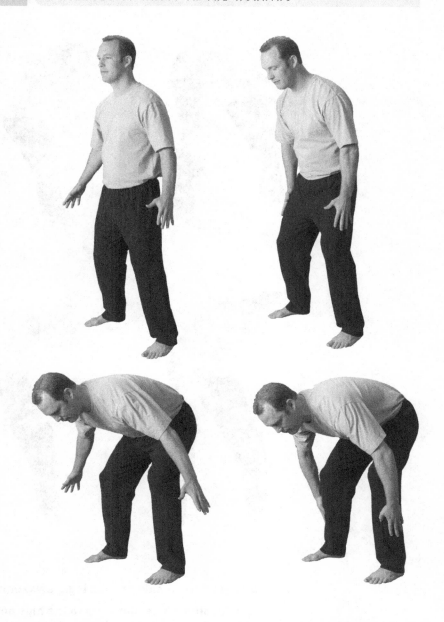

6. Next, slap down the outside of your legs with the palms of your hands. Go all the way down to the outside of your feet and back up.

This stimulates the major lines of energy in the body.

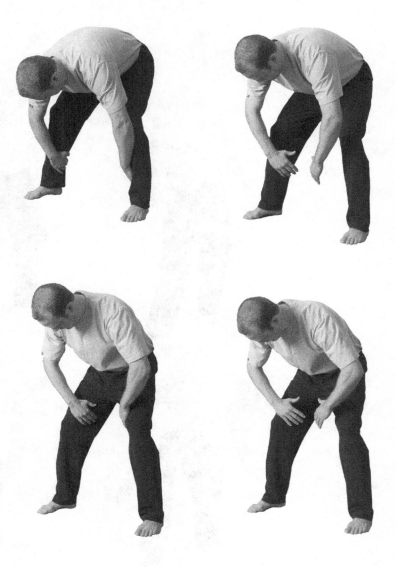

7. Now slap up the inside of your legs, awakening the energy
   lines in the inner legs. Come up to the hips and gently work
   your way through the abdomen to the chest.

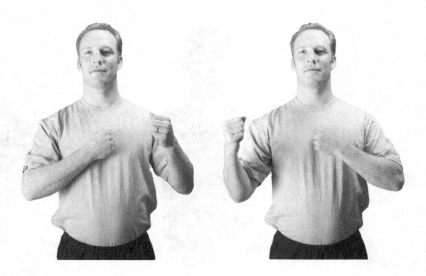

8. Come to standing upright and knock on your sternum and the center of your chest with light fists.

(If it worked for Tarzan it can work for you, too!) This stimulates the lungs, heart, and thymus gland. Stimulating the thymus gland is rejuvenating and can slow down aging.

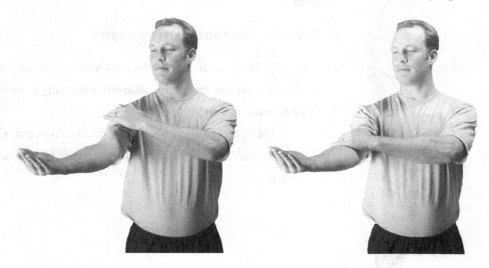

9. Continue by opening your left fist, and slapping the inside of your right arm down to the hand.

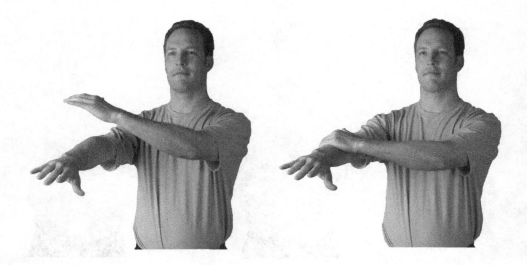

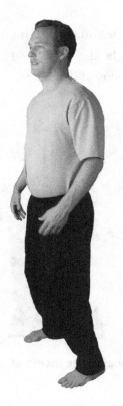

10. **Then slap up the outside of the right arm, through the neck and shoulder area, and back to the chest.**

11. **Switch sides, slapping down the inside of the left arm to the hand, then up the outside of the arm to the neck and shoulder area.**

12. **End by knocking on the sternum again.**

13. **Shaking. Bring your arms down by your sides and start to shake your wrists and arms. Allow the shaking to work up to your elbows and shoulders.**

Think of an Olympic swimmer before an event, shaking out her arms. Athletes do this intuitively to clear tension and energize.

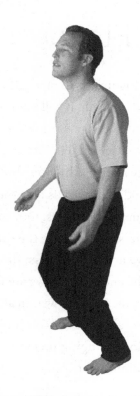

14. Next, begin to bounce lightly into your heels, shaking the entire body.

Feel your spine open. Allow your head, neck, and shoulders to relax. Shake loose any areas where you chronically hold tension.

15. Slowly stop shaking, and bring your hands down to your sides.

Feel the energy buzzing and tingling through your arms, hands, back, legs, and feet. Feel the flow.

Breath Flow

This flow will strengthen the lungs and increase the power of your breath. It will train your body to breathe more deeply throughout the day. By taking more oxygen into the body with each breath, you will increase the body's vitality and energy. The quality and depth of our breath is fundamental to the health of our bodies. Breath is also the key element in clearing stress and balancing emotions. Our breathing reflects how we feel. When we are sad or crying, the breath comes in spasms and gasps. When we are under stress, the breath becomes shallow and locked in the chest. When we are feeling good, the breath becomes deeper, calmer, and slower. In all meditation traditions, the breath is used to calm the mind. Think of this next flow as a moving meditation, bringing precious energy to the body, clearing stress, and calming the mind.

1. **Holding Up the Sky.** Standing with your feet shoulder width apart, bring your arms in front of your abdomen with your palms facing up.

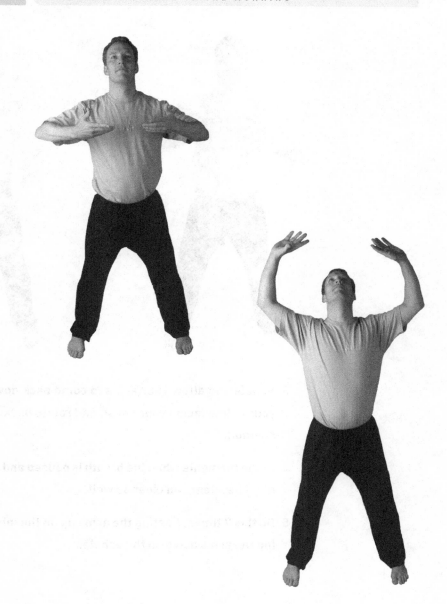

2. Inhale and slowly bring your arms up, palms facing the chest, and then float your arms up over your head, turning your palms to face the ceiling. At the same time, look up to the ceiling. Pause at the top of the inhale.

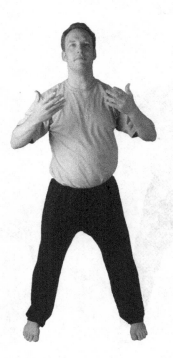 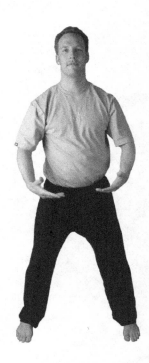

3. Exhale and allow your arms to come back down, again with your palms facing your chest, and rotate back to the starting position.

4. At the moments when the breath is paused and silent, let your mind be silent and clear as well.

5. Do this 7 times, floating the arms up on the inhale, and floating the arms down on the exhale.

Mind Flow

Setting your intention for the day might be the most important internal exercise yet. We have all heard how powerful the mind is, but rarely do we tap into this potential. Creating the day and life we want comes from the quality of our awareness. Flexibility is as important as setting an intention, since life often buffets us with unexpected winds and storms. This next flow teaches us to keep the intention on our purpose firm while adapting to life's constant changes.

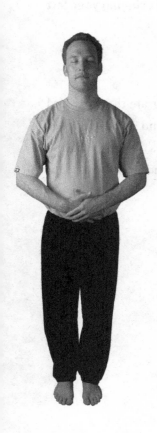

1. **Bamboo in the Wind. Bring your feet close together and place your hands over your lower abdomen.**

2. **Take a few deep breaths into the belly.**

3. **Relax into your legs. Feel your body like bamboo in the wind, gently rocking back and forth or left and right.**

4. **Like the bamboo, feel rooted into the ground but flexible in your mind and body.**

5. **Take 30 seconds to visualize how you want your day to go. How do you want to feel throughout your day? Bring in sights, sounds, and sensations.**

6. **From this place of inner strength and flexibility, set your intention to have a wonderful and rewarding day.**

More Magic for Energy

1. **Centering. Keep your feet shoulder width apart. Stand tall, lifting your head toward the ceiling.**

2. **Bring your left hand under your abdomen, palm facing up. Take a deep breath and circle your right hand down to your side, then back and around behind your body.**

3. **Exhale, and bring your right hand down the midline of your body, toward your lower abdomen.**

4. **Repeat on the other side, circling your left arm down and around on your inhale, then exhaling and bringing your left hand down the midline of your body.**

5. **Go back and forth 3 times on each side.**

Centering is an energetic exercise to integrate the body and mind. Throughout the week we get depleted and give out a lot of energy to work, family, friends—the necessities of life. Centering is a way to fill back up. It helps bring the mind into the present moment and renew the body-mind system.

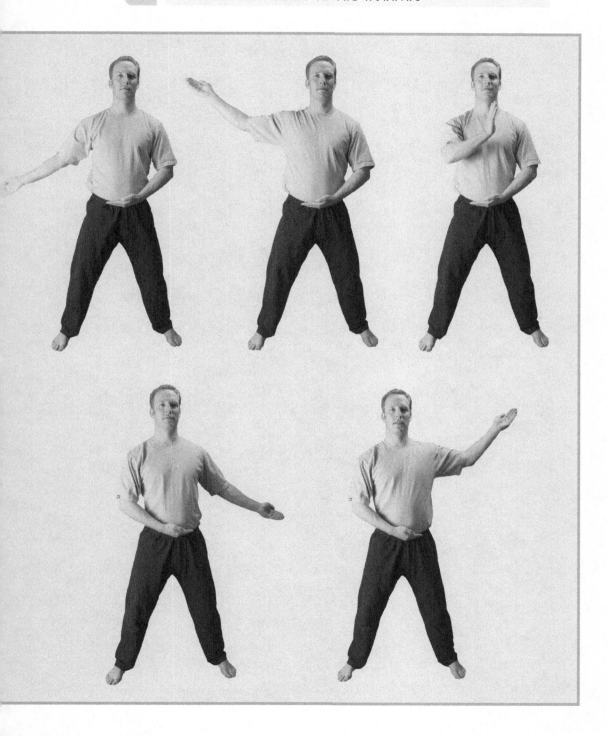

4

7 Minutes of Magic in the Evening

The evening routine helps get you in tune with the natural rhythm of the night. Allowing the stress and challenges of the day to be released is vitally important to a clear mind and a healthy body. Stress becomes detrimental when it stays with us day after day. Think of a sun setting into the ocean, the peace and tranquility of day transforming into night. This is the quality of energy we want to cultivate with our evening routine.

The evening flow clears stress and tension, cultivates calming and relaxing energy, and prepares the mind and body for sleep. The holistic health-care model emphasizes letting go of negative emotional energy and stress from your body and mind before going to bed. This evening routine is specially designed to release pent-up tension so that you can unwind and relax.

What most of us don't realize is that we need energy to sleep. This is a different quality of energy than the morning energy. The sleeping process is very complex; the mind is processing the thoughts of the day and purging emotional energy through dreams. The body is cleansing and detoxifying from the day and repairing cellular damage. This all takes a great deal of energy. Without energy, you can't do everything that you need to do while you sleep. This routine will give you the relaxed energy you need both to unwind at the end of the day and to get deep, nourishing rest throughout the night.

Spinal Flow

The Spinal Flow is a great exercise for clearing stress and tension from the back. Regarded as a spinal cord enlivening exercise, this movement facilitates the flow of spinal fluid through the back, creating suppleness. To clear the physical and mental tension of the day, the spinal cord is vitally important. Mental tension needs an outlet, and by synchronizing the spinal movement with deep breathing, mental stress is distributed through the nervous system and cleared out through the body.

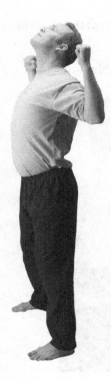

1. **Spinal Cord Breathing. Begin by bringing your hands up in front of your shoulders. Inhale, arch your back, and look up.**

2. **Next, on an exhale, round your back and tuck your tailbone under. To do this, you can squeeze your buttocks as the tailbone comes under.**

3. **Inhale, open your chest, and look up.**

4. **Exhale, round your back, and tuck your tailbone under again.**

5. **Go back and forth, feeling all the joints in the spine moving and tension releasing through the central nervous system. Do this 7 times in each direction.**

Upper Back and Neck Flow

The Upper Back and Neck Flow clears tension from the muscles in the neck and shoulder area. As we go through the day, we collect tension in this area of the body. With stress, work, and a hurried lifestyle, tension accumulates and our shoulders slowly start to grow toward our ears. These muscles then get shorter, spasm, and contract, causing pain and stiffness. Holding tension in the neck and shoulders takes a lot of energy. Think of contracting the muscles in your arms all day; you would be pretty tired after a few hours. Well, this is what is happening in the neck and shoulders—we are unconsciously contracting these muscles all the time. As you go through this sequence, feel the tension melting like ice in the hot sun.

1. Palm Press Behind Back. Bring your palms together behind your back, fingers facing down.

Find a place where you feel comfortable—the hands don't have to be very high.

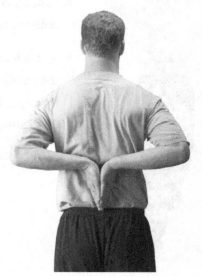

2. **Now gently circle your head, bringing your left ear toward your left shoulder. Let your head fall forward, chin toward the chest. Then rotate to the other side, right ear toward the right shoulder.**

This movement stretches the sides of the neck and the trapezius muscle; extends down through the forearms; and opens the joints in the neck. Be careful not to bring your head too far back. Bringing the head too far back puts pressure on the cervical spine. Just bring the head up to a neutral position, then to the side, down, to the other side, and back to neutral.

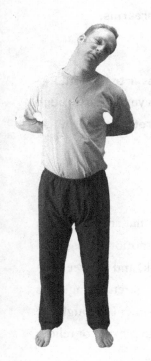
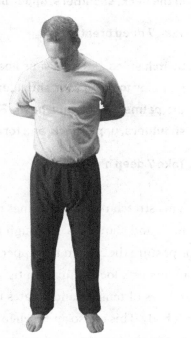
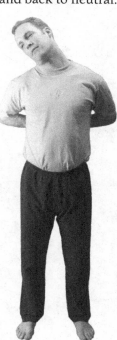

3. **Circle your head slowly and feel the muscles stretch, keeping your palms pressed together so you can feel the stretch all the way down through your wrists.**

4. **Repeat in the other direction, circling your head 7 times in each direction.**

More Magic for the Neck

1. **Shoulder Stretch. Take both hands out to the sides and press your palms downward, as if you were trying to reach the floor.**

2. **Spread your fingers and flex your wrists upward. Consciously bring your shoulders down as you press through the palms.**

3. **Next, gently lean your head over to your right shoulder. Relax your head as you lean it; don't use force. Feel the stretch in the neck, shoulders, upper back, and forearms.**

4. **Take 7 deep breaths.**

5. **Switch sides and lean your head gently over to the left. Remember to bring your shoulders down as you press through the palms. Relax your head. Feel the stretch in your neck, shoulders, upper back, and forearms.**

6. **Take 7 deep breaths.**

This stretch releases the lines of tension that accumulate in the neck and shoulders. Through repetitive motion, stress, and poor posture the area in the upper back, neck, and between the shoulders gets locked up with tightness. This stretch lengthens these lines of tension and creates better alignment through the upper body. This is also an excellent exercise to prevent or relieve tension in the forearms and wrists.

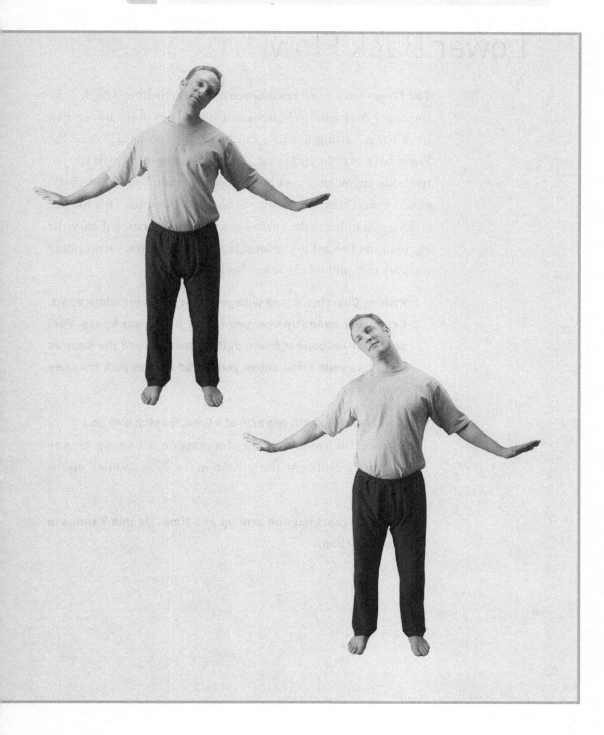

Lower Back Flow

The Lower Back Flow releases tension from the lower back. Like the upper back and neck, tension accumulates in the lower back from stress, sitting too long, and working too hard. When the lower back is tight and tense, it creates tension through the entire body. If you have ever had lower back pain, you know that it affects everything; even walking becomes difficult. This routine is designed to bring the spine back into alignment, enhance the circulation of blood to the muscles, and stretch the surrounding muscles that pull on the lower back.

1. **Picking Cherries. Stand with your feet shoulder width apart. Bring your hands up over your head. Bend your knees. Feel as if your tailbone is being pulled down toward the floor as you raise your arms above your head as if to pick cherries from a tree.**

2. **Next, reach up with one arm at a time. Stretch way up.**

   Feel the lower back muscles elongate. This is a great way to equally distribute the tension in the back and line up the spine.

3. **Continue reaching one arm up at a time. Do this 7 times in each direction.**

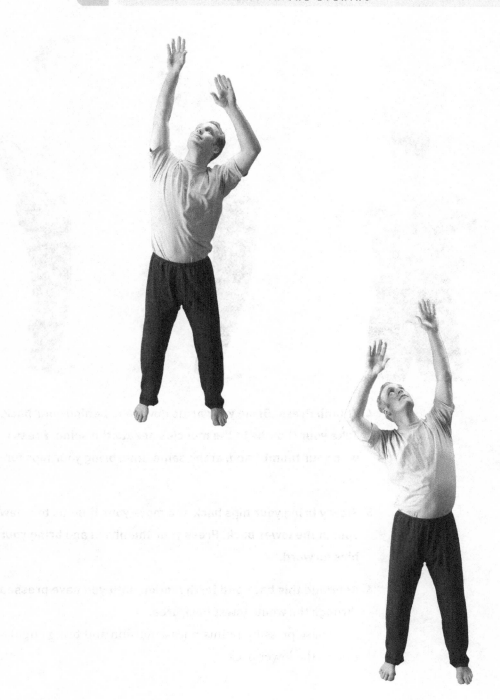

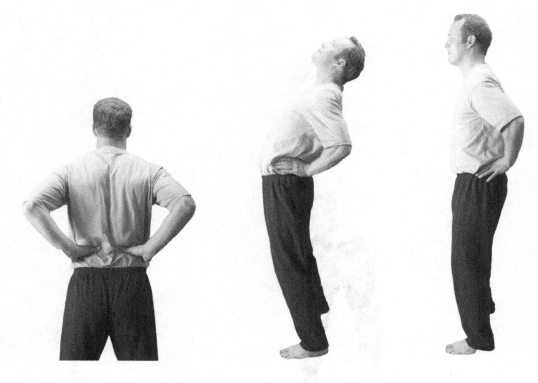

4. **Thumb Press. Bring your arms down and behind your back. Take your thumbs to the muscles next to the spine. Press in with your thumbs and, at the same time, bring your hips forward.**

5. **Slowly bring your hips back and move your thumbs to a new spot in the lower back. Press your thumbs in and bring your hips forward.**

6. **Continue this back and forth motion until you have pressed through the whole lower back area.**

These pressure points release tension and bring circulation to the lower back.

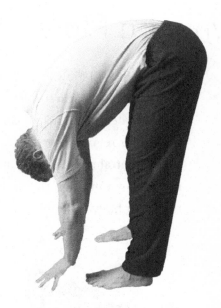

7. Forward Bend. Bring your arms in front of you and hang forward. Don't force the stretch. Simply relax forward with the knees slightly bent, and feel the hamstrings stretch. Hold the stretch for 7 seconds. If you want a stronger stretch, straighten your legs.

Tension in the hamstrings is directly linked to the lower back. Feel the line of tension from the hamstrings to the lower back start to release and lengthen.

Downward Flow

The Downward Flow is the next step in unwinding and releasing pent-up tension from the day. After being upright all day, this part of the sequence will help rebalance and transition your mind and body into relaxing for the evening. This flow focuses on the spine, central nervous system, and hips, a progression from the mind, down through the upper body, and finally releasing into the lower body.

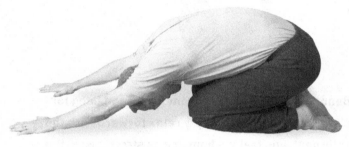

1. **Child's Pose. Bend your knees and bring your hands to the floor. Then step back with both feet and bring your knees to the floor, moving your buttocks toward your heels and extending your arms out in front of you.**

   Child's Pose is a natural posture for rejuvenating the body and mind after a long day. It is not a strong stretch, but it has many benefits for the system such as releasing tension from the back and calming the nervous system.

2. **Keep your arms extended out in front of you and press into the floor with your arms and hands, bringing your hips back even farther.**

   Feel the extension through your upper back and the release through your lower back.

3. **Hold this posture for 7 deep breaths.**

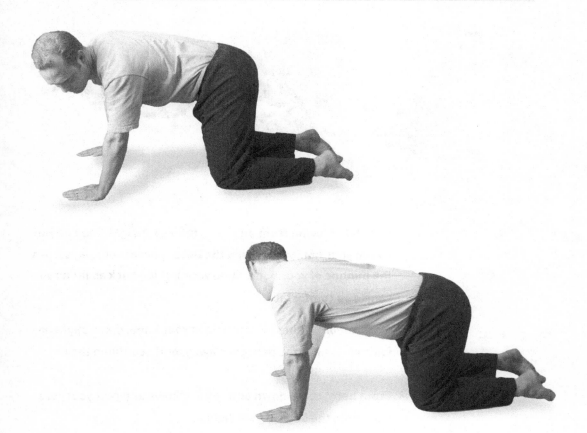

4. Dog Wagging the Tail. Come up onto all fours. Begin to move your tailbone and lower back side to side.

How often do you get to flaunt your best side? This exercise moves the spine in a lateral motion, releasing tension from those large muscles that run up the back and support the spine.

5. Allow the movement to move up your back to your neck and shoulders. Feel all the joints moving.

6. Wag the tail for 7 seconds.

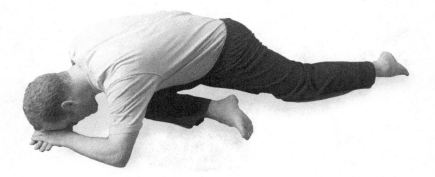

7. **Peacock. Moving from all fours, take your right knee up between your hands and bring the lower part of your leg across the midline of your body. Slide your left leg back as far as you can do so comfortably.**

   Modification: **If there is any pain in your knee, make slight adjustments until the pain goes away, or discontinue the pose.**

8. **From here, come down onto your elbows and rest your forehead onto the back of your hands.**

9. **Breathe into the pose. Feel your body expand on the inhale, and sink deeper into the stretch on the exhale. Relax the weight of your upper body into the stretch.**

   This is an excellent hip opening stretch and is especially good to do at the end of the day. It releases tension from those muscles that get tight from sitting in a chair, car, or airplane.

10. **Take 7 deep breaths.**

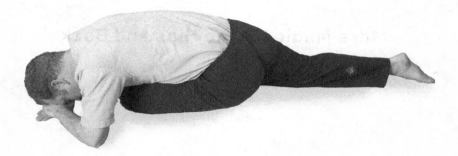

11. **Switch legs by coming back onto all fours, then sliding your left knee up between your hands and bringing the lower part of your leg across the midline of your body. Slide your right leg back as far as you can do so comfortably. Take 7 deep breaths on this side.**

12. **From here, come down again onto your elbows and rest your forehead onto the back of your hands.**

13. **Take 7 deep breaths on this side.**

14. **Roll to the outside of your left hip and bring both legs in front of you, sitting on the floor as a way to move into the next exercise.**

More Magic for the Hips and Back

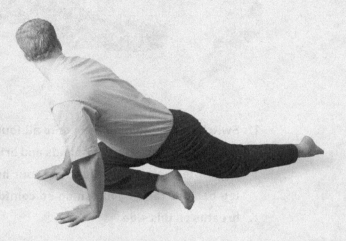

1. **Peacock Looks at Tail. Start on all fours, then take your right knee up between your hands and bring the lower part of your leg across the midline of the body. Slide your left leg back behind you as far as you can do so comfortably.**

2. **Twist and Look at the Tail. Slowly bring your chest down to your right knee. Then, using your arms, press into the floor and turn and look over your right shoulder. Continue to press into the floor until your arms are straight.**

3. **Repeat the movement one more time with your right leg forward.**

    Feel the opening in your right hip and your spine. The twist opens up the line of tension between your right hip and glutes, and into the muscles of your lower back.

4. **Come onto all fours once again.**

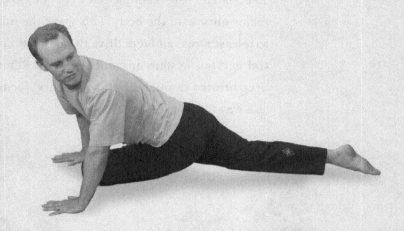

5. Take your left knee up between your hands and bring the lower part of your leg across the midline of your body. Slide your right leg back behind you as far as you can do so comfortably.

6. Slowly bring your chest down to your left knee. Then, using your arms, press into the floor and turn and look over your left shoulder. Continue to press into the floor until your arms are straight.

7. Repeat the movement again with your left leg forward.

Seated Flow

The Seated Flow is simple but dynamic, stretching almost every major muscle in the body. This gives the mind the opportunity to release stress and repetitive thought patterns through the central nervous system and out the body. Remember to take long deep breaths throughout this sequence, focusing on your exhale as a way to clear tension.

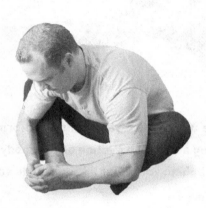 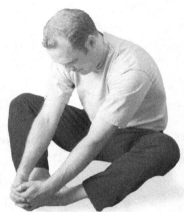

1. **Turtle. Bring the soles of your feet together. Interlock your fingers around your toes and stretch forward.**

2. **Use your hands to gently pull your forehead toward your toes.**

3. **Hold for 7 seconds.**

4. **Next, tuck your chin in toward your chest.**

5. **Allow your back to round, gently pulling your spine back.**
    Feel the stretch in your upper back and neck. This is an excellent stretch for the area between the shoulder blades.

6. **Hold for another 7 seconds with a rounded back.**

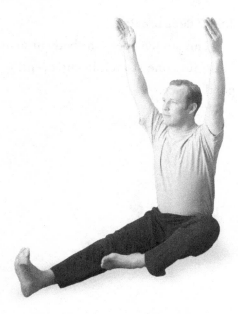

7. **One Knee Bent. Straighten your right leg and leave your left leg bent. Reach up with both hands, bringing them over your head to elongate the spine.**

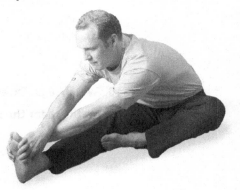

8. **Extend forward and cross your arms around your lower leg or foot, depending on your flexibility, left hand on the outside of your leg or foot, right hand on the inside of your leg or foot.**

   Remember, never push the stretch too far. Just go as far as it feels comfortable to you.

9. Take 7 deep breaths.

This stretch opens the body in so many ways. If you were to do just one stretch in the evening, this one would be a good choice.

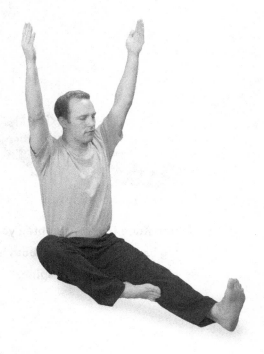

10. Switch legs. Extend your left leg, right leg is bent with the foot resting near the inside of your left knee.

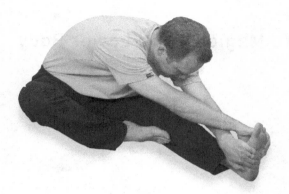

11. Reach both hands up over your head. Extend forward and cross your arms and hands around your lower leg or foot, right hand on the outside of your leg or foot, left hand on the inside of your leg or foot.

12. Take 7 deep breaths on this side.

More Magic for the Lower Body

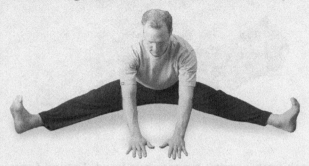

1. **Seaweed in the Ocean. Sit with both legs in front of you as wide as you can comfortably.**

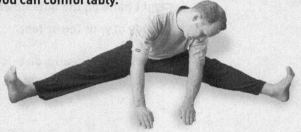

2. **Stretch your arms forward along the floor. Feel the opening in your inner legs, hamstrings, and hips. Take one deep breath.**

3. **Next, feel the stretch in your spine by gently rocking back and forth, left and right.**

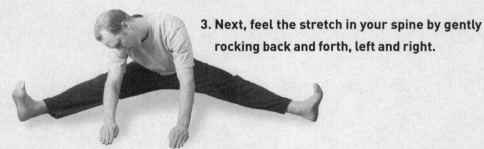

This is a great way to open the legs and hips and release tension in the lower back that is caused by tight hamstrings.

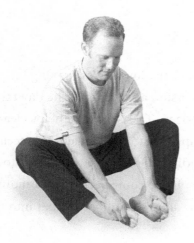
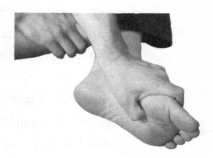

13. **Foot Massage. Bring your left leg in so that the soles of your feet are facing each other.**

Massaging the feet stimulates key pressure points and helps relax the mind, lower blood pressure, and prepare the body for deep, restful sleep. In traditional Chinese medicine it is used for insomnia.

14. **Use your thumbs to massage into the bottoms of your feet. Work the entire area with firm pressure for thirty seconds.**

A particularly good point to massage is just below the ball of the foot. When you curl your toes, it is the area that makes a hollow or a pocket. This point is called Bubbling Springs, and it relaxes and calms the mind.

15. **When you finish massaging your feet, lie down on your back.**

Lying Flow

The Lying Flow continues the journey of moving into rest and relaxation, letting the tension and stress of the day release and preparing the body for sleep. This sequence helps clear tension out of the lower back, hips, waist, and legs, and is especially good after sitting all day. It brings the lower body back into balance, aligning the pelvis and spine to come back into harmony. Taking deep breaths in this flow allows you to go deeper into the poses and feel more connected.

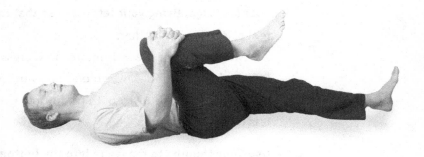

1. **Hug One Leg into Chest. Lie on your back and bring your right knee up toward your chest, allowing your left leg to straighten out onto the floor. Interlock your fingers around the knee and gently pull it in.**

    Feel your right hip and lower back open. You might even feel your hip flexor stretch on the front of the left leg.

2. **Hold for 7 seconds, relaxing into the posture.**

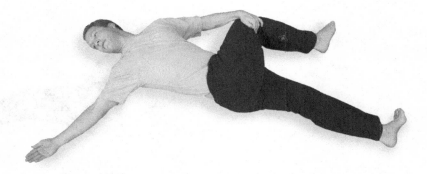

3. **Twist. Take your right knee and cross it to the left over your body and bring it to the floor.**

4. **Hold your right knee down with your left hand and turn your upper body to the right. Your lower body and right leg are to the left and your upper body is stretching in the opposite direction, toward the right.**

5. **Use your breathing to go deeper into the pose. Feel the breath move down through your ribs and into your lower back, allowing the tension to release on the exhale.**

6. **Take 7 deep breaths.**

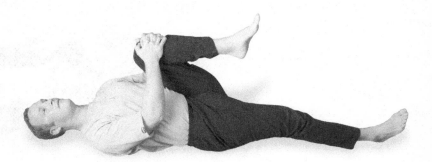

7. Switch legs. Bring your left leg up toward your chest, allowing your right leg to straighten out onto the floor. Interlock your fingers around the knee and gently pull it in.

Feel your left hip and lower back stretch and lengthen.

8. Hold for 7 seconds, relaxing into the posture.

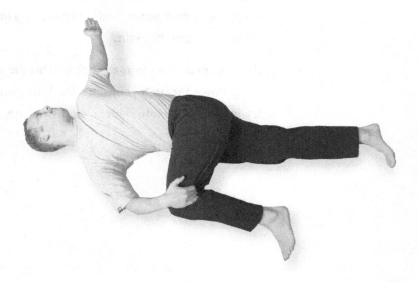

9. Now go into the twist. Cross your left knee over your body and bring it to the floor.

10. Hold your left leg down with your right hand and turn your upper body to the left.

Your lower body and left leg are to the right and your upper body is stretching in the opposite direction, toward the left.

11. Again, take 7 deep breaths.

More Magic for the Hamstrings

1. **Lower Leg Foot Circle. Bring both feet to the floor with your knees bent.**

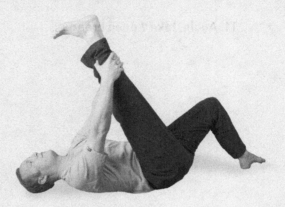

2. **Next, lift your right leg straight up into the air. Hold both hands behind your right calf or knee, interlocking your fingers.**

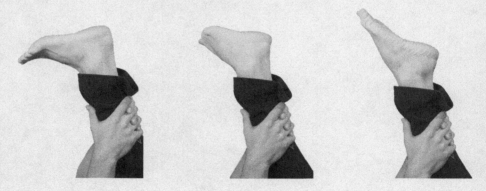

3. **Circle your right foot and ankle, bringing a full range of motion through the joint.**

4. **Circle 7 times in each direction.**

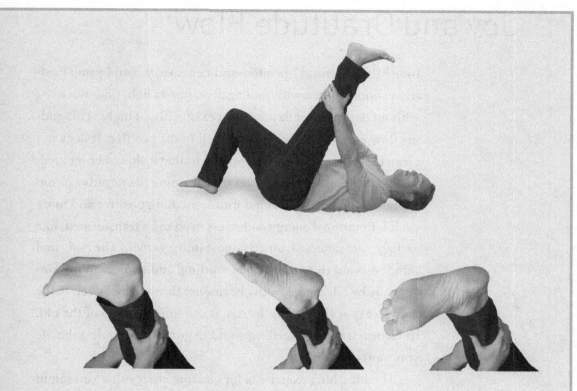

5. Bring your right foot back to the floor, knees bent. Then lift your left leg, interlock your fingers behind your knee, and circle your left foot 7 times in each direction.

This is another dynamic stretch for opening the ankle joint and stretching the calf, shin, and Achilles tendon. When the lower leg is more flexible, you have more stability in your foundation. Having supple, strong ankles, calves, and feet will give your entire body more balance and structure.

Joy and Gratitude Flow

In life there is always positive and negative, yin and yang. Positive cannot happen without negative, just as light does not exist without darkness, or day does not exist without night. This ending flow is about immersing yourself in the positive. It does not mean that the negative does not exist or that it should be ignored. The goal here is simply to start transforming the negative or old energy in the body and mind into something positive and more useful. Emotional energy and stress need to be transformed, like garbage into compost, and compost into a garden. The body and mind respond to gratitude, joy, smiling, and relaxation physiologically by releasing healthy hormones through every cell of the body. Now, at the end of the day, is the time to let go of the old, transform it into the fertile ground to grow and manifest the life you want to live.

The breathing exercise is for clearing energy that you might have picked up or taken on throughout your day. It washes the system from the inside out. In yoga, qi gong, and many other traditions, sounds are used to create a vibration and influence the subtle energy in the body.

1. **Inner Balance Sound. Lie on your back with your hands out to your sides, palms facing up. Take a deep breath in. Feel the abdomen expand first, then the rib cage, and at the top of the inhale, fill up the chest.**

2. **As you exhale, quietly make the sound "Heeeee." This is done in a whisper, not using the vocal cords. It should sound like the wind gently moving through the trees.**

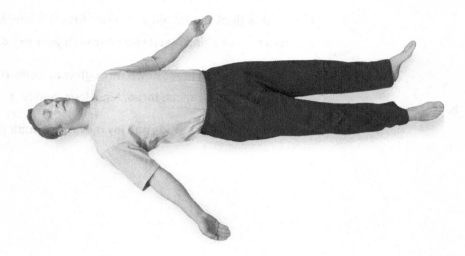

3. **As you make the sound, allow the exhalation to roll down from the chest, through the ribs, and finally squeezing the abdomen back toward the spine.**

4. **Feel tension being released out through your fingers and toes.**

5. **Repeat this 3 times.**

6. **Inner Smile. After you have finished the sound, gently smile.**

   Feel the subtle curving of your lips and the widening of your eyes. You are not posing for a picture. This is an inner smile for yourself, and another way to transform negative to positive, stress into tranquility. There are eighty muscles in the face, and studies have shown that when we smile we actually induce the release of mood-enhancing hormones.

7. **With your mind's eye, visualize a sunset with golden light on the horizon.**

8. Feel this light shining on your face. Breathe it in through the pores of your skin. Feel it wash through your mind.

9. Allow the light to move down through your body, through the neck, shoulders, arms, torso, hips, legs, and feet.

10. Feel a sense of gratitude and joy moving through you.

PART III

Living with More Vitality

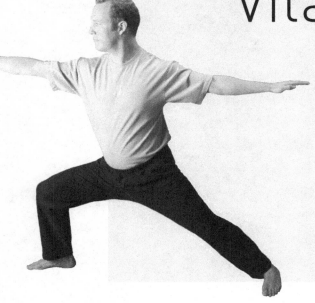

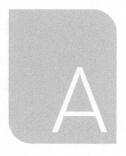

After doing your morning and evening routines, you are still left with twenty-three hours and forty-six minutes. This part of the book offers some simple and effective lifestyle suggestions on how to bring more energy, more health, and more magic into the rest of your life each and every day.

Through your lifestyle choices you control more than 70 percent of how well and how long you live. By the time you reach fifty, your lifestyle will determine 80 percent of how you age. The suggestions and exercises that follow will not only add years to your life, but life to your years.

5

Exercise: Don't Sweat It

Everyone knows that exercise, like eating your veggies, is good for your health. Yet millions of people don't exercise. The modern struggle with weight problems, high blood pressure, anxiety, depression, and chronic low energy are a direct result of a lack of regular exercise. About half of all people who take up a new exercise program abandon it within a few months. The most common reason people quit or never take up exercise in the first place is the lack of convenient exercise opportunities and/or a lack of time.

The 7 Minutes of Magic routines are a strong foundation for your daily workout, but for overall fitness you'll need to complement the program with other forms of exercise. Some people would love to be active for seven minutes, then spend the rest of the day on the couch channel-surfing and only moving their thumb. But the truth is, our bodies are built for physical activity—far more than we get in our modern lives. In addition to these seven-minute routines, getting aerobic exercise should be an important part of your life, even if it is as simple as a fifteen-minute walk.

For decades, scientific studies have affirmed the tremendous benefits of exercise and its key role in health and vitality. Simple exercise routines, like 7 Minutes of Magic, done regularly, provide an incredible variety of physical, emotional, and psychological benefits.

I have two doctors, my left leg and my right.

—George Trevelyan, author and historian, 1913

Think of your workout as powerful medicine. In one of countless examples, scientists at the University of Pennsylvania found that blood flow from exercise fights inflammation in the arteries in the same way a high dose of glucocorticoids, a steroid, would. Inflammation is a prime suspect in heart disease. When blood flows, the receptors in the cells in the lining of your blood vessel are triggered, producing anti-inflammatory effects.

Walking is the nearest activity to perfect exercise.

—Professor J. Morris and Dr. Adrianne Hardman, 1997

Exercise strengthens the muscles, bones, and heart, and even boosts the immune system. Anatomically, it releases beta-endorphins, those pain-reducing, mood-regulating neurotransmitters that lift our spirits and produce temporary euphoria. The general scientific consensus is that exercise enhances physical strength and vitality; improves mood, self-esteem, confidence, productivity, capacity to handle stress, sleeping patterns, and general wellness; and increases longevity. Even on a cellular level, exercise increases the body's supply of mitochondria, which facilitate cell metabolism and conversion of food to usable energy. Increased mitochondria in the cells mean more energy for the body.

Here are some examples of the benefits of exercise:

- **Exercise and Postmenopause:** By exercising regularly, postmenopausal woman can reduce their risk of premature death by 30 percent. Even women who are physically active only once a week are more likely to live longer.

- **Exercise and Body Fat:** The average percentage by which your amount of body fat could increase if you quit exercising for just eight months is 8½ percent.

- **Exercise and Male Sexuality:** Men who don't work out have an increased risk of developing erectile dysfunction.

- **Exercise Versus Diet:** Weight loss achieved through exercise can reduce abdominal fat more successfully than diet alone.

- **Exercise and Insomnia:** People who don't exercise have more trouble falling asleep and staying asleep.

- **Exercise and the Immune System:** Those who exercise less are more likely to contract upper respiratory tract infections.

- **Exercise and Mood:** Regular exercise as a treatment for mild to moderate depression is as effective as and sometimes more effective than individual or group therapy and antidepressant medications. Antidepressant medications often take two to three weeks to become effective and long-term benefits are inconsistent. Exercise has been shown to alleviate depression, often within ten minutes, and to increasingly diminish and even eliminate it over time.

- **Exercise and Longevity:** Exercisers have an all-cause mortality rate (your likelihood of dying) that is less then one-third that of non-exercisers.

Exercise: An Eastern Perspective

It is clear that exercise plays an important role in all aspects of our lives. But from an Eastern perspective, enjoyment is essential to reaping the health benefits of exercise. Just as exercise is good for your physical heart, joyfulness is good for your emotional heart. In other words, you should try to find a form of exercise that is fun and joyful. Why torture yourself and push yourself to do activities that you don't enjoy?

It seems logical that exercise should be enjoyable. With so many ways to move our bodies, why should we force ourselves to engage in activities that we don't like? If you hate jogging but force yourself to do it anyway, your body and mind are not in harmony. In a way, it is like running on a treadmill and eating a bowl of ice cream at the same time. The mind and body need to be aligned in order to create the body and the life that you want. In addition, only if you find joy and satisfaction in your exercise will you be able to sustain your routine.

I've been through every diet under the sun, and I can tell you that getting up, getting out, and walking is always the first goal.

—Oprah Winfrey

In tai chi and qi gong, the "no pain, no gain" attitude does not apply. Often the more pain you have during an exercise, the more pain you'll have after the exercise. In nature, animals don't force themselves to exercise—it is just part of who they are. Notice how children exercise with joy and playfulness. Do not underestimate the fun factor in your workouts.

Think about activities you truly find pleasure in and make time for them. Make a list of all the enjoyable sports, games, and activities you like to do. Plan them into your schedule once or twice a week. This, along with your 7-Minute routines, will deliver the greatest benefits to your body, mind, and spirit.

Exercise and Nature

Whenever possible, you should try to exercise in nature. Exercising outside offers a wide variety of benefits that working out indoors doesn't provide. Hiking, jogging, mountain biking, playing on the beach, or working in the garden all offer your body fresh air and energy from the trees, woods, and landscape. Fresh air has more vital energy than the air indoors.

This is especially true of locations with trees or large bodies of water, because negative ions are much more plentiful in these areas. Negative ions are absorbed into the body and energize the system. All exercise is beneficial for clearing stress, but exercising outdoors is more restorative and emotionally balancing.

Have you ever noticed that when you are walking along the beach or hiking in the forest, you feel better? Spending time in nature is emotionally purifying. We exhale carbon dioxide, our body's exhaust, and the trees absorb it. They in turn give off oxygen, which we inhale to stay alive. In the same way, nature can recycle and transform our negative emotions and refresh us in a way that only the best therapy session can match. Whenever possible, take your physical activity outside and draw in nature's precious energy and life-sustaining vitality.

The Magic of Walking

How much would you pay for a miracle pill, taken each day, that would lessen your chances of developing breast cancer by 20 percent, heart disease by 30 percent, and diabetes by 50 percent, and would help you live longer and healthier into old age? Let's just say that it would be more popular than Viagra. That miracle pill is walking. Lace up your walking shoes and you will reap all of these health benefits.

Walking is one of the best forms of exercise. It is a magical workout because of its simplicity and tremendous benefits. It can be done practically anywhere at any time, by nearly anyone, regardless of physical condition, and it does not require elaborate facilities or equipment.

Walking produces results both in short-term fitness and in long-term health equal to any other aerobic exercise—including jogging. Jogging has tremendous health benefits, but walking has all the same benefits without the wear and tear on the body. When you jog, you land with three or four times your body weight. When you walk, you land with only one and a half times your body weight. This is especially important for the joints.

Walking is the ideal aerobic exercise, bringing oxygen to the blood and every cell in the body. As with the 7 Minutes morning routine, when you walk, you use your body's large muscles, which pump circulation through your entire blood stream, increase metabolism, and energize your whole body.

Exercise research shows that walking four miles burns more fat than running the same distance in less time. Walking is an excellent aerobic exercise. It keeps you fit and it helps you take off extra weight and keep it off. Obesity has become an epidemic among Americans and other people in the industrialized world, and it is especially troubling that so many children are now overweight or obese. Lack of exercise is a major factor, and walking is an important part of the solution. Here are some of the health benefits of walking:

- Improves circulation

- Helps breathing

- Combats depression

- Bolsters the immune system

- Helps prevent osteoporosis

- Helps prevent and control diabetes

- Controls weight

- Reduces the risk of coronary heart disease and stroke

- Lowers blood pressure

- Reduces high cholesterol and improves blood lipid profile

- Reduces body fat

- Enhances mental well-being

- Increases bone density, helping to prevent osteoporosis

- Reduces the risk of colon cancer

- Reduces the risk of non-insulin-dependent diabetes

- Helps flexibility and coordination, reducing the risk of falls

Multiple studies have shown that people are most likely to stick to an exercise program when it is part of their daily lives. Walking is ideal because you can incorporate it into many activities you would be doing anyway. Once you start looking for opportunities to walk, you will be amazed at how many there are. Here are a couple of examples:

- Park ten minutes away from where you want to go.

- Take the stairs instead of the escalator or elevator.

- Walk to lunch.

- Walk to a park and eat your lunch.

- Walk after dinner.

Although walking by itself has tremendous benefit, I am going to teach you a form of walking, Tai Chi Walking, that delivers even more benefits and will make every step count the most for your health and your happiness. Here's how it's done.

Tai Chi Walking Practice

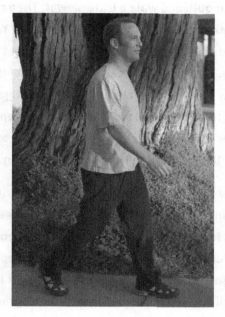

Tai Chi Walking does not mean doing slow and graceful tai chi moves or making martial arts sounds as you karate chop your way through downtown. As you will see, Tai Chi Walking is a simple, effective way to use your breathing to increase lung capacity while focusing your mind as you stroll.

Your Tai Chi Walking practice should be done three or four times a week for twenty to thirty minutes. As I've said, walking can be done almost anywhere—around the block, down the street, near your office, in a park, along the beach, or, my favorite, in the woods. Make time, wherever you are, to take advantage of this life-extending practice.

1. **Establish your pace. Find a pace that best suits you, not too fast and not too slow. You want your walking practice to feel vigorous and invigorating.**

2. **Use your arms as you walk. Pump the arms with your stride. This will activate the muscles in the upper body. Using the arms will make walking more powerful and effortless.**

3. **Breathe through your nose during the entire walk. The breath should be pulled in and out through the nose. The breath is deep, rhythmic, and vigorous, but not too quick. Keep your breath full and long; this will deliver the greatest benefit. Breathing in and out through the nose will strengthen the**

lungs, filter the air, stimulate the production of endorphins, and increase energy. If you feel out of breath at any time, exhale out through the mouth and walk a little slower. Then resume the deep breathing in and out through the nose. You should feel the breath at the back of your throat, both on the inhale and the exhale. In tai chi, this is called the Breath of the Tiger. It is also widely used in yoga, and is often called Ujjayi breathing. (See chapter 6, "Breathing," for a more in-depth explanation of the benefits of breath work.) This vigorous breathing separates Tai Chi Walking from simply strolling.

4. *Tai Chi Walking is also a form of meditation,* and it helps bring the mind to the present moment. By entering into the present moment, the mind is focused on what is in the here and now, not the past or the future. This is a good way to reset your mind and get out of habitual ways of thinking, and it will increase the psychological benefits of your exercise program. This mental focus makes Tai Chi Walking feel quite different from letting your mind simply meander.

5. Getting your mind and thoughts present can be challenging. The simplest, most effective way to do this is to use your senses. Start with sight. *Notice what you see.* Don't force yourself to look around; simply notice—the blue sky, the clouds, the ocean, the trees, the cars, the other people. Root your mind into your visual sense. Stay with what you are seeing for 3 to 4 minutes.

6. Then, *tune into your auditory sense.* Notice what you are hearing—the birds, the wind, the rhythm of your feet. Anchor your mind into the present moment through listening. Focus on your sense of hearing for 3 to 4 minutes.

7. Next, *get in touch with your kinesthetic sense.* Observe what you are feeling—your feet making contact with the ground, the air moving in and out of your lungs, the wind blowing through your hair, the warmth of the sun caressing your face, the air moving through your fingers. Bring your mind into the moment by feeling sensations in your body. Do this for 3 to 4 minutes.

8. After separating each individual sense, *try experiencing all your senses at the same time.* This can be challenging, but with a little practice it can be a wonderful expansion into the present moment. Open your mind and observe sight, sound, and touch all at once. To do this you have to relax and allow your mind to be reflective like a still mountain lake.

9. Whenever your mind wanders, bring your attention back to your breath and back to your senses.

10. Continue with this deep-breathing, mind-expanding walking practice for about 20 minutes.

6

Breathing: The Bridge Between Your Mind and Body

The benefits of working with the breath are profound in many ways. The way you breathe directly influences the quality of your life. In fact, the way you breathe might be the most important factor in how you feel.

Think about how you breathe when you are sad or crying. You inhale with short, shallow gasps and exhale with either long wails or choppy sobs. If you are angry, in breaths are usually constricted and out breaths are long and forceful. Under stress, the breath can actually become so shallow that it appears almost nonexistent. On the other hand, when you are feeling good, the breath is calm, deep, and even. The amazing thing about breathing exercises is that they can make the relationship work in the reverse; by changing the way you breathe, you can also change the way you feel.

Try this: Look up, and take a really deep breath, filling up your belly, ribs, and chest. Smile, and say out loud, "I am so depressed." As you might have noticed, this exercise is fairly comical. What's even more interesting is the fact that it is almost impossible to breathe deeply and feel depressed while holding an expanded posture. In a great study done on depression, one group took antidepressants drugs, and the other group simply had to look up, smile, and breathe deeply periodically throughout the day. The smiling group had even better results than the group on drugs. How we hold our body powerfully affects how we feel. If you want to feel better, breathe more deeply and smile more. Remember that breathing is a reflection of thought and emotion, the bridge between the mind and the body.

Breath unleashes the vital energies of life. Inhale fully to be inspired and take in more of life; exhale completely to expire the old and no longer useful out of the body. This process refreshes the system in every moment, clearing out stagnant emotions and thoughts and taking in the new possibilities with each breath. If we cannot inhale completely, psychologically we cut ourselves off from new experiences, adventures, and creativity. If we cannot exhale completely, we hold on to the past and are weighed down by old emotional hurts and wounds. To breathe is to be alive. To breathe deeper is to delve into life more fully.

Think of your breath as Vitamin O, oxygen being the most important nutrient that you take into your body. These are some of the benefits of deep breathing:

- Energizes the entire system

- Provides cells with sufficient oxygen for optimal functioning

- Clears stress and tension from the muscles

- Supports the lymphatic system to cleanse the blood

- Detoxifies the blood

- Massages the internal organs for better functioning

- Increases lung capacity for more energy

- Calms the mind

- Facilitates communication between the conscious and unconscious mind

- Acts as a bridge between the mind, body, and spirit for balance, harmony, and spiritual growth

- Promotes health and healing

- Increases communication between the left and right hemispheres of the brain, stimulating both sides of the brain at the same time

- Helps harmonize the nervous system and reduce stress

- Increases fundamental vitality

- Deepens meditation

- Expands consciousness

Chronic shallow breathing drains energy and allows stress to take root in the body, resulting in tight muscles and tension. Most of us are unaware that our respiratory systems are chronically constricted. In fact, medical researchers believe a lack of oxygen in the system is the prime cause of 1.5 million heart attacks each year.

Shallow breathing underoxygenates the blood, organs, muscles, glands, and all the cells in the body. Deep breathing helps take pressure off the heart. Deep diaphragmatic breathing acts like another pump to circulate blood more efficiently through the body.

Shallow, constricted breathing overworks the heart, suffocates the brain (15 to 20 percent of the oxygen goes to the brain), weakens the immune system, and leads to disease and premature aging. Many catastrophic illnesses have their roots in chronic underoxygenation caused by chronic shallow breathing. Underoxygenation leaves toxins in the blood that are then recirculated throughout the body. Dr. Otto Warburg, winner of a Nobel Prize for his cancer research, explained that cancer had only one prime cause—the replacement of normal oxygen restoration for the body's cells by oxygen-deficient respiration. Deep breathing increases oxygen to the cells, which is one of the most important factors in living a disease-free and energetic life. As Dr. Warburg said, when cells get sufficient oxygen, cancer will not and cannot occur.

Oxygen is our most essential food, the fuel that ignites the essential bodily processes—everything from digestion and assimilation to hormone secretion to numerous brain functions.

Mouth Breathing
Versus Nose Breathing

In qi gong, there is a saying, "The mouth is for eating, the nose, for breathing." This seems fairly intuitive, yet the majority of us are sucking in air through the mouth. Energetically, we are not making use of the amazing health features of the nose. The nose is the body's primary defense against germs, impurities, dust, and bacteria entering the lungs, the bloodstream, and the body. The nose has bacilli-fighting glands, mucous membrane passages, and thousands of filtering hairs to protect the body. The mouth has none of these protective features, and allows a virtually unprotected passage directly into the lungs.

When you breathe through the mouth, there is a tendency to fill only the chest. When you inhale through the nose, the breath naturally penetrates the body more deeply. Try taking a deep breath through the mouth and notice where you feel the expansion. Now, take a slow deep breath through the nose. Did you notice how the breath is drawn deeper into the body when inhaling through the nose, expanding into the lower abdomen? Breathing through the nose engages the diaphragm, and is the most natural, healthy way to breathe. Watch the way babies and children breathe: their abdomens and rib cages naturally expand and contract.

Though the lungs have a total air capacity of about 5,000 milliliters, the average breath is only about 500 milliliters. But we can learn to inhale much more air than we normally do—with the proper breathing techniques, we can almost double our breathing capacity, taking in twice the amount of energy per breath.

The proper functioning of every cell in our bodies depends upon the quality of our breathing. Breathing is the dance of life, uniting all living things in a necessary symbiotic life-support system. We live on the exhaled oxygen of plants; plants live on our exhaled carbon dioxide. Every breath reveals interdependence with the environment. We live in an ocean of energy. Life offers each of us a full portion of vitality. Why decline this abundance of life force through shallow breathing? Why breathe just enough to get by, when you can breathe deep enough to truly thrive?

Magic Breathing, the Wave Technique

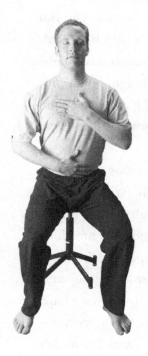

Think of the tide of the ocean lapping up onto the shore. The water rolls in, pauses, then returns to the ocean. Between the incoming and outgoing tide there is a lull—a stillness before movement. This is how we should breathe, mirroring the movement of the tide. As you will soon experience, the movement of the breath flows through the entire torso like a wave in the ocean. The breath starts in the lower abdomen, then rises up through the ribs and crests in the chest. On the exhale, the wave of movement descends back down—from the chest, through the ribs, and down into the abdomen. Try it for yourself.

1. **Find a comfortable position, either sitting up with a straight spine, or lying face up on a comfortable surface. Sitting is preferable and keeps you more alert, but lying down works well, too.**

2. **Bring your right hand over your navel and your left hand on the center of your sternum at the center of your chest.**

3. **Take a deep breath in through your nose. Feel your lower abdomen expand first.**

4. **As you continue to inhale, let the breath rise up through the ribs.**

5. **Keep inhaling until the breath reaches your upper hand at the chest.**

6. **Exhale through your nose.**

7. Feel the breath relaxing and descending from the chest.

8. Allow the breath to move down through your ribs.

9. At the end of the exhale, allow your abdomen to move back toward your spine as you squeeze the breath all the way out.

10. At the top of the inhale, allow the breath to pause for one or two seconds.

11. At the bottom of the exhale, allow the breath to pause once again for one or two seconds. A pause in the breath is like the lull of the tide and creates balance in the mind and energy in the body.

12. Continue taking full, deep breaths.

13. Take at least 7 breaths. You will start to feel the benefits almost immediately. If you can do this exercise for 7 minutes, the benefits will be even greater.

7

Food: Chew More, Eat Less, Lose Weight, Live Longer

From low fat to low carb, from South Beach to Okinawa, there are countless diets and nutrition books on the market, all advocating a different program. In this section, I want to give you a refreshing perspective: Just as important as what you eat is how you eat. What I want to explore with you is how the process of eating plays a vital role in metabolism, vitality, and nutrition. The more skillfully you eat, the less you have to worry about what you eat. Just as we need to learn what to eat, we also need to learn how the process of eating influences metabolism.

There really are lots of reasons to eat—the taste, social engagements, your mother told you to, and of course, because you're hungry. It doesn't necessarily matter what your reasons are; the ultimate goal is to fuel up your body with energy. This section is about tuning into the process of eating so that we not only enjoy our food more, but we also get more energy out of the food we eat.

In the last decade alone, nutritionists, doctors, and diet and health "experts" have written hundreds of books promoting dozens of dietary theories and routines. For the purposes of this book, let's highlight some key points that are universally agreed on and move on to a refreshing way to look at how we fuel our bodies—how we eat food.

Here are some commonsense dietary suggestions:

- Eat a balanced diet of protein, complex carbohydrates, and healthy fats.

- Eat whole grains, complex carbohydrates (such as brown rice and whole-grain bread) rather than simple carbohydrates (such as white rice and white bread).

- Eat fresh organic fruits and vegetables.

- Don't overeat.

- Eat when you're hungry.

- Minimize junk food and processed foods.

- Drink plenty of pure water every day.

- Get essential fatty acids from fish or nuts.

- Drink green tea.

- Get plenty of antioxidants from fresh fruits, vegetables, legumes, herbs, and spices.

People are obsessed with diets, for a good reason. Obesity cuts millions of lives short and can wreak havoc on our overall health and energy. Yet our weight, health, and energy levels are more than just the food we eat. Why is it that over 80 percent of diets don't work and that the weight people lose is usually back within a year?

There are many reasons diets fail—some diets are difficult to incorporate into everyday life, some limit our food choices and are not sustainable, and others don't take individual needs into consideration.

With so many diets failing, there is a refreshing and simple Taoist solution to loosing weight and getting healthy: Chew more.

Rather than continually changing the food we eat, jumping from one diet plan to another, just chew more. Most of us chew our food an average of only seven times before swallowing. Throughout most of this book, seven is a great number, but here is where it doesn't apply. If we chewed each mouthful twenty to thirty times, our average caloric intake could be cut from more than 3,000 calories per day to 2,000. And we would feel full on less food. Chewing more allows digestion to begin in the mouth and prepares the entire digestive system.

The Taoist recommendation for healthy eating is "Drink your food." That means, chew your food so thoroughly that it becomes liquid in your mouth. This helps digestive enzymes in the saliva begin to break down the food and prepare the body for assimilation. By the time the food gets to the stomach, the work is already partially done. In this way, we get more energy and more nutrition from the food we eat. Also, the internal organs work better because the digestive process is more efficient.

Chewing more means eating more slowly. It generally takes twenty minutes to realize how full you are. If you rush through a meal, you almost always overeat. When you eat slower, you enjoy your food more and you eat less. And chewing more increases your metabolism so you burn more fat.

Chewing Meditation

In this practice, you want to chew your food about twenty to thirty times. While you are chewing, bring your attention to the process of chewing and how the food tastes and feels in your mouth. It is important here to try not to do other things, like watch television, drive, or read. It is much better to have all of your awareness on the process of eating. Pay close attention to every bite. Food eaten mindfully will be easier to digest, and you will be less likely to overeat.

1. **Sit down for your meal.**

2. **Take a few deep breaths.**

3. **Take a bite of something delicious.**

4. **Chew 20 to 30 times.**

5. **Savor the food.**

6. **Feel the texture in your mouth.**

7. **Notice the taste and flavors.**

8. **Have the intention that what you are eating will deliver energy and vitality to your entire body.**

8

Water: Replenishing Your Source

Proper intake of water is a magical part of a balanced diet. It is so simple, so essential, that many of us are missing its amazing benefits. Water is the source of all life—we come from it and are literally made of it. Taoists have always emphasized the importance of water as a key factor in our energy and health.

We evolve from conception to birth as human beings by floating in a sea of amniotic fluid. A developing fetus is initially 99 percent water. At birth we are 80 percent water. As we age, our percentage of water declines. Most adults are about 70 percent water. Our brains are 85 percent water, and even our solid bones are 25 percent water. As we age even more, we are reduced to 50 percent water, and even less when there are health issues and disease.

Inflexibility and stiffness get more pronounced as we age, and prevent us from living life to the fullest. Staying flexible, with the 7 Minutes of Magic program and adequate hydration, is vitally important for a youthful body.

Every function of the body hinges on the efficient flow of water. Every cell requires regular daily hydration for health and energy. The distribution of water ensures that hormones (the chemical messengers in the body) and nutrients get transported to the proper place. Chronic lack of hydration creates problems for every part of the body. From the individual cells to the gross tissues, from the muscles to the bones, and from the internal organs to the brain, the proper amount of water is an absolute necessity.

Many studies link chronic underhydration to depression, chronic fatigue, fibromyalgia, ulcers, headaches, asthma, allergies, high blood pressure, compromised liver function, urinary infections, constipation, bad breath, and obesity. You might have noticed that doctors recommend drinking plenty of water for almost any ailment.

Water is the cheapest form of medicine. Without proper hydration, we may find ourselves in a downward spiral. When a person is dehydrated, water may be rerouted from various places in the body, for example, from the cartilage in the joints to the internal organs, creating pain and stiffness. The pain in the joints keeps us from exercising or moving our bodies properly. We can then become sedentary, overweight, and lethargic.

Water is the only liquid that cures underhydration. Soda, tea, and coffee do not count as water and actually can be mildly dehydrating. If the majority of your beverages are coffee and soda, dehydration can be a real problem. Pure water is the best hydrating element.

Not only do the Taoists say to "drink your food," they also recommend that you "chew your liquids." This means to taste your liquids and meditate on how they cleanse the system and give life, energy, and vitality. As you drink, feel the water transforming into your body—becoming your cells, organs, muscles, and bones.

Warm Beverages Versus Cold Beverages

In Chinese medicine, drinking cold liquids is discouraged. I am not going to dissuade you from an ice-cold glass of water or a cold beer on a warm summer evening, but there is good reason to drink room temperature beverages whenever possible. Cold drinks take energy to warm up, which drains energy from the digestive system. Whatever you eat or drink will be warmed to body temperature. If you drink a room-temperature beverage or warm beverage, it is easier on the digestion and doesn't take energy to heat it up. If it is hot outside, you can drink more cooling beverages without adverse effects on digestion. But when it is cold out, it is especially important to drink warming beverages. Try this: During at least one meal every day, sip tea or warm water with lemon rather than a cold beverage, and see how you feel afterward.

A Simple Way to Stay Hydrated

Your body needs a minimum of six to eight 8-ounce glasses of water a day to stay hydrated. This does not include coffee, tea, or soda. These drinks all have a dehydrating effect. In fact, if you drink coffee, it is a good idea to drink an extra 8-ounce glass of water just to balance the coffee's dehydrating effects. The best time to drink a full glass is thirty minutes before any large meal. Drinking too much during a meal dilutes the digestive enzymes and makes it harder to assimilate food properly. And, as I've already mentioned, it is best to sip warm liquids during your meal rather than gulp down ice-cold beverages.

9 Meditation: Coming Back to Your Center

When some people think of meditation, they imagine an old man sitting under a tree with a loincloth and a long beard in search of enlightenment. Or some think of meditation as boring, an impractical waste of time in our modern world. Whatever your thoughts are about the subject, I want to spark your curiosity and explain to you the numerous and practical benefits meditation can have in your daily life. This section of the book will show you how meditation can be one of the most rewarding and health-supportive activities in your daily routine. It will also give you a simple 7-Minute Meditation.

Think of meditation as a mini-vacation from the fast-paced, intense, emotionally draining world we live in. It is a journey, an inner journey where you will discover peace, tranquility, and a state of deep relaxation.

Meditation is an exploration of your own inner potential. We all want more energy, greater health, deeper understanding, more joy, and greater fulfillment. These qualities already exist. You don't have to create them. Meditation is a practice of unwinding and coming back to a place of being centered and balanced. It is a natural remedy, a form of relaxation that benefits the mind-body system in myriad ways.

The purpose of this section isn't to go into the history of meditation or the countless techniques developed over the centuries, but to distill meditation into a practical technique that will give you more energy and reduce your stress. It is as simple as that.

Meditation offers dozens of scientifically proven benefits. According to the ancient Eastern traditions, the real cause of stress and suffering is not what happens to you, but how your mind responds to what happens to you.

In the East the incessant chatter in the mind is often referred to as "monkey mind." The analogy compares the mind to a monkey swinging uncontrollably from branch to branch—from idea to idea, from plan to plan, from this memory to that, from thought to emotion—without ever calming down. This mental turbulence leaves little room for creativity or intuitive thinking. In fact, psychological research indicates that about 95 percent of the thoughts we have today are the same thoughts we had yesterday. Meditation moves us beyond the habitual mental patterns and opens our minds to a deeper potential that we all have within.

Mind-body medicine reiterates what Taoist sages and yogis have been telling us for millennia—your body and your mind form one seamless and inseparable whole. When your thoughts keep leaping like the proverbial monkey from worry to worry, your body responds by tightening and tensing. Over time, this contraction creates stagnation in the energy system that eventually leads to pain and disease.

Meditation is simple but requires discipline. Calming the mind is elusive, like grabbing at water and watching it slip through your fingers.

As our 7-minute routines remind us, the more you reconnect with your deeper self, the more you infuse your body and mind with life energy and healing. And as researchers have proven again and again, this life-giving energy mobilizes your body's healing resources, bolsters your immune system, and naturally facilitates the process of repair and renewal.

Meditation has been used for thousands of years as a way to tap into the innate healing capacity of the body and mind. By allowing the body to move into a state of deep relaxation and the mind to enter into a calm and clear space, the entire system returns to a state of equilibrium. Meditation is focused relaxation, the dynamic balance between tranquility and being full of energy.

Why spend seven minutes or more of your limited free time each day to quiet your mind and deepen your breath? You could be lifting weights, jogging on a treadmill, or surfing the Internet. Here are seven good reasons:

- **Rejuvenating the Body:** Meditation can lower blood pressure, release stress from the muscles, and ease tension.

- **Calming the Mind:** An agitated mind inevitably produces emotional turbulence and stress in the body. As the mind settles, relaxes, and opens during meditation, stress evaporates from the system.

- **Experiencing Present Moment Awareness:** Getting connected to the beauty in the here and now, stepping out of the hustle and rush from one activity to another, allows for deeper meaning and balance.

- **Improving Relationships:** Meditation can help you feel more connected with others in positive, meaningful ways.

- **Experiencing Flow:** Meditation helps you get in a zone where you feel connected to your sense of purpose. Meditation helps you delve into the space of effortlessness, that place where life flows joyously.

- **Creating Balance:** Meditation can be a means of creating harmony and a feeling of being centered and grounded. Life can be chaotic, stressful, and full of change. Meditation is a way to discover harmony amid the chaos.

- **Enhancing Performance:** Studies have shown that basic meditation practice alone can enhance perceptual clarity, creativity, self-actualization, and many other factors that contribute to superior performance.

The paradox of meditation is that although it might seem inconsequential, it can bring about so many amazing benefits. In our modern lifestyle, our bodies may feel perpetually braced against the next challenge, making it extremely challenging to relax and enjoy life. Meditation can provide a simple but powerful antidote. Meditation gives you the inner resources to deal with difficult circumstances and the stress these situations evoke. Meditation practice elicits a state of balance and tranquility, allowing you to shed problems and slough off stress like old skin.

How Meditation Heals

To begin with, meditation, like many of the techniques in this book, is preventative. By teaching you how to relax your body and calm your mind, meditation helps you to avoid getting sick in the first place. Meditation restores balance and harmony within by slowing the mind, regulating the breath, and focusing the intent.

Most physicians recognize the relevance of psychological factors and the importance of relaxation and stress reduction in maintaining health. In fact, the emerging field of mind-body medicine developed in the 1970s when scientists studying the abilities of Eastern-trained meditators witnessed that the mind could have an extraordinary effect on the body. More recently, researchers studying immune response have shown that the immune system and the nervous system are inextricably intertwined and that psychological and emotional stress can suppress immune function, encouraging the growth or spread of immune-related disorders such as cancer and autoimmune diseases.

Herbert Benson, a cardiologist and professor of medicine at Harvard Medical School, coined the term "Relaxation Response." Benson pioneered the field of mind-body medicine with the publication of his bestseller *The Relaxation Response* in 1975. Benson studied meditation and how it induces relaxation. Participants in this meditative state would experience a bodily response of relaxation, and the benefit was a reduction in stress through the counteraction of the fight-or-flight response. In subsequent studies, Benson found that the Relaxation Response had a beneficial effect on reducing hypertension, headaches, heart disease, alcohol consumption, anxiety, and PMS.

The autonomic nervous system, which regulates vital internal processes, becomes more stable, integrated, and adaptable from meditation, as indicated by its increased ability to recover rapidly from the effects of stress.

The body of research into the benefits of meditation is extensive and cross-validated from many sources. For example, the finding that Transcendental Meditation (a type of meditation using a mantra) programs decrease stress is validated by physiological changes such as decreased cortisol levels (the major stress hormone), decreased muscle tension, normalization of blood pressure, increased autonomic stability, and increased EEG coherence. At the same time, a variety of psychological changes also indicate a reduction in stress, including decreased anxiety and depression, decreased post-traumatic stress syndrome, and increased self-actualization.

Research published in the *International Journal of Neuroscience* has also found that meditators in their mid-fifties have a biological age twelve years younger than their chronological age. This means that if you are fifty-five years old, your body would be functioning as if you were forty-three years. As I mentioned before, aging is accelerated by stress. By minimizing the wear and tear caused by stress, meditation promotes both good health and greater youthfulness.

The 7-Minute Meditation

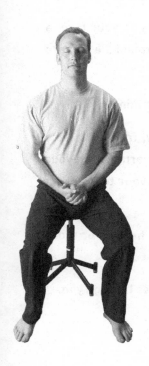

The 7-Minute Meditation is designed to give you maximum results in the least amount of time. You can set a timer if you want to be exact or just have the intention that you will meditate for seven minutes. Commit to doing nothing more than sitting quietly, doing this visualization, and watching what happens. Don't pick up the phone, don't answer the doorbell, don't add another item to your to-do list. Just sit, breathe, and observe how your body responds to the guided imagery.

This guided visualization comes from a Taoist meditation technique called the Inner Smile. This technique adds to the many benefits of meditation by eliciting a subtle smile on the face, which engages the eighty or so muscles around the eyes, jaw, and temples, sending positive energy through the body. Whenever you smile, a positive, healing message is sent through the body. Think of the Inner Smile as a way to awaken the dormant healing energy in the body and the mind.

1. **Sit comfortably in a chair or on the floor.**

2. **Lift through the top of your head so that your spine is straight and tall.**

3. **Bring your hands on top of your knees or bring your palms together in your lap.**

4. **Relax and take a few deep breaths.**

5. **You can incorporate some of the Wave breathing (see pages 167–168) throughout this meditation.**

6. Imagine that you are watching a sunset. Golden light is streaming toward you and shining on your face.

7. Feel this light bringing an uplifting quality to your face, a smile between your eyes and very slightly around the corners of your mouth.

8. As you breathe in, draw this image into your mind.

9. Visualize this light permeating your body, from your face down your neck, from your neck down your arms, from your arms down through your torso, and from your torso down your legs.

10. Direct golden light to wherever you need healing or more energy.

11. Continue breathing deeply as the light moves through you.

12. Continue for 7 minutes.

10 Sleep: Don't Go to Bed Too Tired

I n Eastern medicine, there is a saying: *Don't go to sleep when you are too tired.* This may seem counterintuitive—if you are tired shouldn't you just go to sleep? You should, but before diving into bed there are a few simple techniques done right before bed that will ensure that you get more deep rest. According to Eastern philosophy, when you are too tired, you don't have the energy to fully recharge while you are sleeping. In this section, I will teach you some simple ways to get the most out of your sleep.

Sleep is an intricate process of infusing the body and mind with rest. Yet while we are sleeping there is a tremendous amount of activity. Think about it—when we sleep we breathe deeply, sometimes deeper than during heavy exercise. Why? Because the body and mind are doing so many things—processing emotions, detoxifying, bringing the system back to equanimity. This all takes energy. If we are depleted, exhausted, we don't have the energy to internally manage these important bodily functions.

A well-rested mind and body can face the challenges of life more effectively. But there is more to sleep than most people realize. Think of a good night's sleep as a way to recharge and fill up with life force. Sleep provides you with an opportunity to reinvigorate every system in the body; it gives you the ability to cope with stress and ward off infection. Sleep gives your body and mind time to regroup, rejuvenate, and rediscover the resilience of balance within.

Stress, physical ailments, and the increasing complexity, tensions, and demands of modern life can interfere with our sleep cycles. A 2002 National Sleep Foundation poll suggested that some 30 to 35 percent of adult Americans experience recurring, chronic, or occasional insomnia. That is about 40 million Americans who are chronically ill with various sleep disorders and an additional 20 to 30 million who experience intermittent sleep-related problems. The consequences of sleep disorders are diverse, serious, and often catastrophic. Common daytime effects of insomnia include low energy, fatigue, difficulty concentrating, impaired memory, diminished motor skills, anxiety, irritability, and being socially off balance. All areas of life, from work to play, from health to emotional balance, are affected by a lack of sleep. Sleep deprivation is an epidemic in our culture.

The Sleeping Pill Dilemma

Sleeping pills can cause morning hangovers and can lead to dependence. They reduce REM sleep, alter normal sleep patterns, and prevent deep rest, often leaving you with less energy during the day. Sleeping pills can also cause "rebound insomnia," meaning that you might have trouble sleeping after you stop taking the pills. In some cases, however, sleeping pills can be very effective. I recommend that most people try more natural methods before taking sleeping pills. Here are some tips on dealing with insomnia:

- Limit television or movies before bed, especially suspenseful shows.

- Reduce your caffeine, sugar, and alcohol intake.

- Get regular exercise.

- Get at least a half-hour of sunlight every day.

- Take a walk after dinner.

- Take a hot bath or shower.

- Keep light and sounds out of the bedroom.

- Do the 7 Minutes of Magic evening routine.

People today spend 20 percent less time sleeping than people did a hundred years ago. This is not surprising considering that we live in a world that is continually awake and on the go. How can we get deeper rest while spending less time in bed?

What should you to do when you are overtired and exhausted? Sleep is the solution, but we want to create better, more restful sleep. To do so, first practice the 7 Minutes of Magic evening routine to give the mind and body relaxed energy for sleep. Then do the simple breathing exercise that follows—it will seduce the body and mind into a state of deep relaxation so you can get more rest and nourishment from your sleep.

The Magical Sound for Deep Sleep

This breathing and meditative practice is part a qi gong exercise routine called the Six Healing Sounds. It is designed to create energy for deep, restful sleep. In Eastern medicine, the emotional energy of the heart directly influences the quality of our sleeping. To have deep, restful sleep, the heart needs to be balanced. The heart is considered to be the king of our emotions. If the heart energy is imbalanced, it leads to turbulent emotions and an agitated mind. When the mind and emotions are in a state of unease, it is difficult to sleep. Have you noticed how busy your mind can be when you have had a stressful or emotionally draining day? These are the nights that it is most difficult to fall asleep or the nights when you might wake up before morning.

This exercise is designed to clear residual emotional energy from the day and promote deep relaxation.

1. **Lie face up in bed and get comfortable.**

2. **Bring your hands to your sides, palms facing up.**

3. **Notice how your body feels.**

4. **Set a clear intention before you sleep. Say to yourself, "As I sleep tonight, allow my body to be recharged and renewed; allow my mind and emotions to be rejuvenated and cleansed."**

5. **Take a few deep breaths and relax into any areas that feel tight or tense.**

6. As you take another deep breath in, fill up the belly first, then the rib cage, and then allow the breath to move into the chest.

7. Exhale and make the heart sound. The heart sound is "Hawww," and is done in a whisper. It sounds like you are saying the word *hot* without the *t* at the end.

8. Again, take a deep breath in, then exhale with the "Hawww" sound.

9. As you make the sound, feel the stress and worries of the day being cleared out of your body and mind.

10. Feel a wave of relaxation moving from the top of your head all the way down to the tips of your toes.

11. Make the heart sound 7 times.

12. After you finish the exercise, simply go to sleep as you would normally.

More Sleep Magic:
The 7-Minute Power Nap

There are numerous benefits to taking naps, which is why many cultures around the world take naps in the afternoon. A midday snooze follows the rhythms and cycles of nature and allows the body and mind to recharge for the rest of the day. The body seems to be designed for napping, as most people's bodies naturally become more tired in the afternoon, about eight hours after waking up.

Studies show that twenty minutes of sleep in the afternoon provides more rest than an additional twenty minutes' sleep in the morning. So instead of hitting that snooze button three or four times, try getting up and doing your 7-minute practice in the morning and taking a seven-minute power nap in the middle of the day.

The optimal nap time is under thirty minutes. Sleeping longer gets you into deeper stages of sleep and makes it difficult to wake up. The minimal power nap time can be as little as . . . yes, good guess, seven minutes. Even a brief rest has the benefit of reducing stress and promoting relaxation. It will give you much more energy for the rest of the day and help you be more productive.

Medical research is confirming what Winston Churchill, Albert Einstein, and Napoleon Bonaparte knew, and what many creative artists are aware of: When you start to fade, nothing beats a nap to recharge the body and mind.

A power nap is a short nap, which means it should be between seven and twenty minutes. You do not want to go into a deep sleep, because your brain will remain sleepy and you will feel groggy.

A brief nap is perfect because it allows you to stay in more shallow levels of sleep, which are very refreshing and can help improve memory, creativity, and productivity. In a 2002 Harvard University study conducted by Drs. Alan Hobson and Robert Stickgold, researchers found that within the first few minutes of sleep, people started to relax and experience brain wave patterns that refreshed them.

There are long-term benefits to napping as well. Naps reduce the chance of heart attack and stroke, and lower stress levels. Studies at Stanford University Medical Center in 2006 showed that people who napped had a 30 percent lower incidence of heart disease. Here are some power nap tips:

- Give yourself permission to nap. Don't feel guilty.

- Remember all the performance, mood, and health benefits you gain by taking a nap.

- Surround yourself with items that make you feel comfortable and calm.

- Use an alarm clock or timer so you don't slip into a deep sleep or worry about when you'll wake up (which makes it hard to relax).

- Nap consistently at the same time every day, even if it's just a quick rest.

- Put your feet up or lie down.

- Set the intention that you will close your eyes and rest for seven minutes, and then feel refreshed and recharged when you wake up.

11

7 Minutes of Magic for Health and Vitality: Bonus Routine

This 7-minute bonus routine is simple and easy but delivers many benefits, including better health and enhanced vitality. The beauty of this routine, like the morning and evening routines, is that it can be done anywhere, wearing any outfit, and it doesn't require using any props. This routine is different from the others in that it is practiced standing, making it easy to do for those who have a difficult time getting on the floor or when you are in a place where getting on the floor wouldn't be comfortable. You can even do these exercises while sitting, which makes for a perfect break from working at your desk. If you do these exercises while sitting, simply focus on the steps that involve the upper body while keeping your feet firmly rooted on the floor.

This bonus routine cultivates inner balance—the combination of both energy and relaxation, so it is a convenient routine to do in the morning, middle of the day, or evening. Inner balance leads to greater health, increased vitality, and deeper relaxation.

The movements are simple flows, which create harmony in the body and mind. Slow, fluid movements train the body to move with relaxation, releasing tightness by training the muscles to let go of habitual tension.

During this routine, remember to focus on relaxation and deep breathing. Allow your body to move like water; keep it fluid and flowing, relaxed and effortless.

Deep Abdominal Breathing

Practicing deep abdominal breathing is one of the best ways to dramatically improve your health in a short amount of time. This exercise will help to repattern your breathing so you will breathe deeper throughout the day without thinking about it. Deep breathing directly influences the quality of energy in your body. As you breathe into your lower abdomen, the center of your body, you will send a message to your body to release stress and tension and bring more vitality to all of your internal organs.

1. **Place both hands over your lower abdomen.**

2. **Relax your chest and breathe into your lower abdomen.**

3. **Feel your belly expand on the inhale.**
   As your abdomen expands on the inhale, the diaphragm moves down and brings more oxygen into your lungs. The downward movement of the diaphragm also brings circulation to the internal organs.

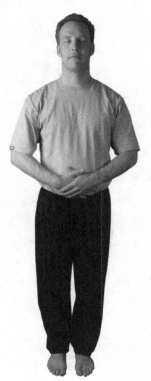

4. **Allow your belly to relax on the exhale. Then, at the end of the exhale, continue to squeeze out any remaining air.**

5. **Repeat, taking 7 deep breaths into your lower abdomen and relaxing on the exhale.**

Spinal Cord Breathing

This is a great exercise for clearing stress and tension out of the back. It is a spinal cord enlivening exercise—the movement facilitates the flow of spinal fluid through the back and thus enhances spinal suppleness. By synchronizing the movement of the back with deep breathing, the joints in the spine become much more flexible. A healthy spine is a key component of a healthy body.

1. **Make loose fists with your hands and bring your arms up above your shoulders.**

2. **Arch your back and look up.**

3. **Next, round your back, tuck your tailbone under, and look down. To do this, you can squeeze your buttocks as the tailbone comes under.**

4. **Do this 7 times slowly in each direction, going back and forth and feeling all the joints in the spine moving and tension releasing through the central nervous system.**

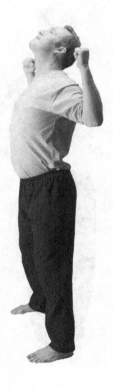

The Wave

The Wave is another excellent spinal movement that creates greater flexibility in the spine and releases tension from the nervous system. During this exercise, think of your spine moving like water—fluid, flowing, and supple. This will enhance the flow of spinal cord fluid in all of the joints in the back and create greater flexibility.

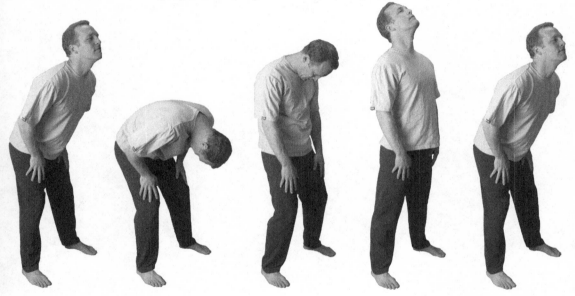

1. Stand with your feet shoulder width apart and place your hands on the front of your thighs.

2. Slightly bend your knees. Inhale.

3. Extend your chin out and move your upper body forward on an exhale.

4. Next, round your back and bring your chin in toward your chest, keeping your knees slightly bent.

5. Roll up like a wave through your spine on an inhale. As you roll up, tuck your tailbone under. When you tuck the tailbone under, the hips move forward.

6. Keep pressing the hips forward until you come all the way back up to standing.

7. Extend the chin again, and repeat the entire exercise 7 times. Think of drawing a big circle in the air with your chin as you do this exercise.

Neck, Shoulder, and Arm Stretch

This is an excellent stretch for releasing the lines of tension that accumulate in the neck, shoulders, arms, and hands. Through repetitive motion, stress, and poor posture, the area in the upper back, neck, and between the shoulders gets locked up with tightness. This stretch lengthens the lines of tensions and creates better alignment through the upper body.

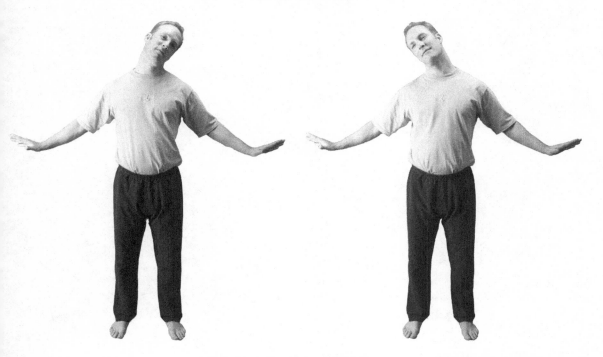

1. **Take both hands out to the sides and press your palms downward, as if you were trying to reach the floor.**

2. **Spread your fingers and flex your wrists upward. Consciously bring your shoulders down as you press through the palms.**

3. Gently lean your head over to your left shoulder. Relax your head; don't use force. Feel the stretch in your neck, shoulders, upper back, and forearms.

4. Take 7 deep breaths.

5. Bring your head gently to the right side. Remember to bring your shoulders down as you press through the palms.

6. Take 7 deep breaths.

Bear Swimming

This exercise is specifically designed to open the upper body by stretching the tendons in the upper back, neck, and arms, by bringing circulation to tight muscles between the shoulder blades, and by increasing lung capacity. Remember to synchronize the breath with the movement and focus on being fluid, like you are moving through water. The motion in this exercise is similar to the breast stroke in swimming. Make sure you move through the chest and upper back to get the maximum benefit.

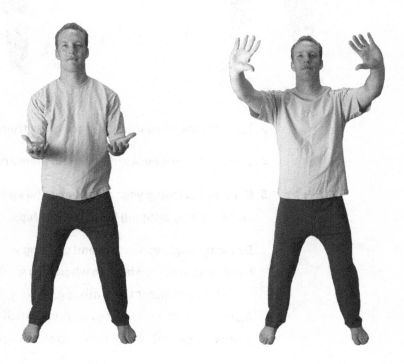

1. **Start with your palms face up in front of your hips.**

2. **Move your hands forward and away from you until your arms are almost straight.**

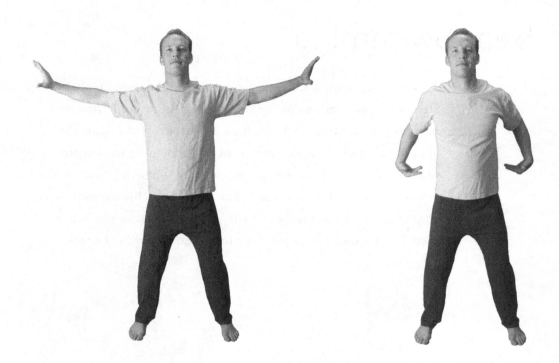

3. **Turn the palms so that they face away from you.**

4. **Open your arms outward and circle them around to your sides.**

5. **Continue bringing your arms back and spiral your hands and arms inward, bringing them by your hips.**

6. **Spiral through, expanding and opening your chest, until your hands and arms are back to where you started—by your hips.**

   The movement is continuous, so try to keep it flowing. Again, it's like swimming the breast stroke. This will bring more energy and circulation into the lungs.

7. **As the arms go forward and away from you, exhale. As you exhale, sink your chest. This will open the upper back and the area between the shoulder blades.**

8. As the arms circle and come back, inhale. As you inhale, expand and open your chest. This will bring more energy and circulation into the lungs.

9. Repeat 7 times.

Return to the Mountain

Return to the Mountain is another flowing movement that brings more energy into the body, while also balancing your emotions and calming your mind. The name of the movement signifies a return to a place of inner tranquility and relaxation. You can use the movement as a way to clear stress, nervous tension, anxiety, or any negative emotional energy.

1. Start by bringing your hands upward from your hips and crossing your wrists with your palms facing toward you.

2. On an inhale, bring your arms up to your shoulders with the wrists still crossed.

3. Next, on an exhale, slowly let your hands and arms spread apart and gently bring your arms back down. As you bring your arms down, feel any old or negative energy leaving the body and mind.

4. You can bring your legs into this movement by bending your knees as your hands come down and standing straighter as your arms come up. Bend your knees as deep as you can do so comfortably. The deeper you bend your knees the more you will work the muscles in your legs.

5. Repeat this movement a total of 7 times.

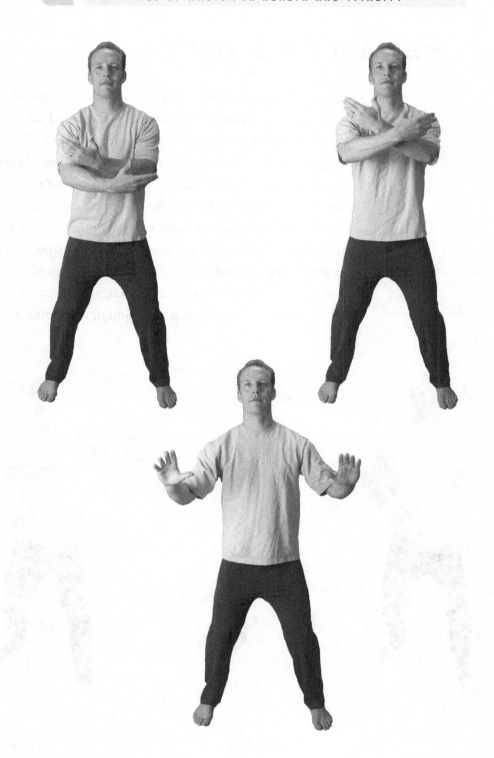

Parting the Clouds

Parting the Clouds is a flowing exercise that strengthens the legs and the foundation of the body. It's designed to keep you grounded and build energy from the legs upward. The feet are staggered with one foot in front of the other in a tai chi stance.

This exercise is also an excellent moving meditation. The name of the movement is a metaphor for clearing out old energy and thought patterns that limit you so you can manifest the life you want to have. As you go through the movements, you can visualize whatever qualities you want to bring into your life. For example, if you want more energy, better health, or more emotional balance, just keep that intention in your mind as you do

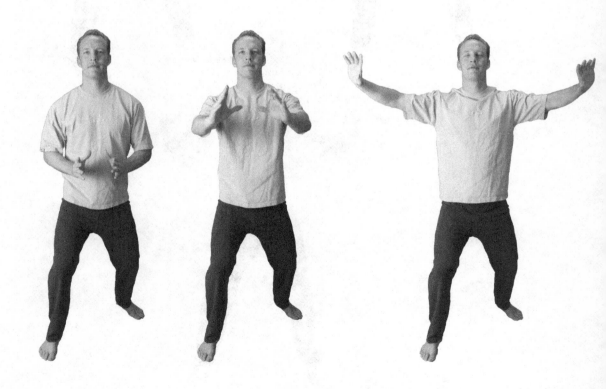

the movements. You can also visualize manifesting whatever else you want: a new job, a new house, more abundance, or a joyful relationship.

1. **Step back with your left foot. Bring both hands in front of your abdomen with the palms facing each other.**

2. **Shift your weight forward slightly, bringing your hands and arms forward.**

3. **Next, turn your palms to face away from you and then circle your hands out to your sides.**

4. **Bring your hands from the sides back in front of your lower abdomen with the palms facing each other.**

5. **Repeat the movement 7 times.**

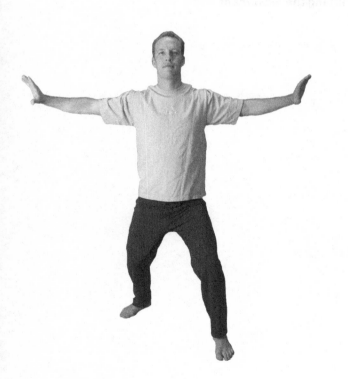
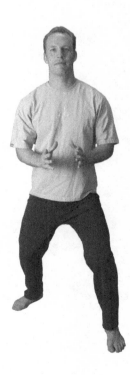

6. Remember to shift your weight back and forth with the movement: as the arms move forward the weight shifts forward; as the arms move out and back, the weight shifts back. The movement should be continuous and fluid.

7. Exhale as you move your hands away from you and forward.

8. Inhale as you circle your arms around and back to the abdomen.

9. Breathe deeply and visualize clearing out any energy that you no longer need in your life (parting the clouds). As your arms open, visualize bringing in the quality of energy that you want to manifest in your life.

10. Repeat on the other side, stepping back with the right foot and continuing the movement.

Centering

This exercise will help you feel more grounded and balanced. It is a flowing movement with an emphasis on pulling energy inward. There are many situations in life that pull us out of our center—work, relationships, driving, standing in line, and all the rest of life's small and large challenges. Centering is a way to fill yourself back up with positive energy. It helps bring the mind into the present moment and renews the body.

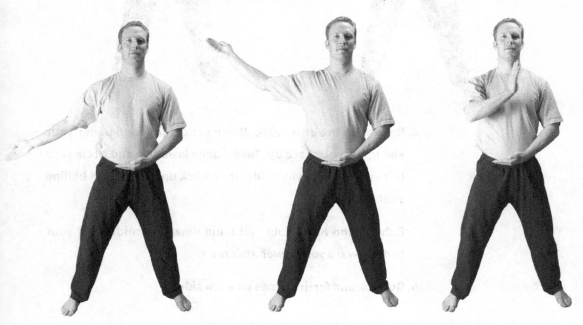

1. **Stand tall, and lift your head toward the ceiling.**

2. **Bring your left hand under your abdomen, palm face up. Take a deep breath in and circle your right hand down to your side, then back up and around behind your body.**

3. **Exhale, and bring your right hand down the midline of your body, toward your lower abdomen.**

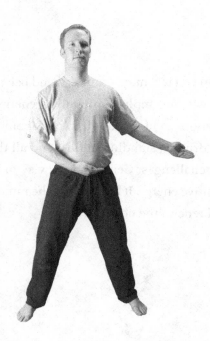
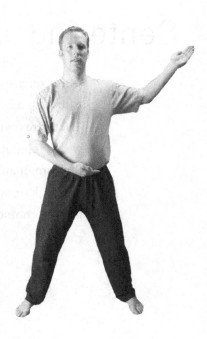

4. Repeat on the other side. Bring your right hand under your abdomen, palm face up. Take a deep breath in and circle your left arm down to your side, then back up and around behind your body.

5. Exhale, and bring your left hand down the midline of your body, toward your lower abdomen.

6. Go back and forth 7 times on each side.

Bamboo in the Wind

This is a deeply relaxing exercise, an excellent way to unwind and come back to a place of inner balance and harmony. The breathing is the same as in the first exercise in this series: deep abdominal breathing. The routine has taken you full circle, ending the same way you started, with a renewed sense of energy, vitality, and relaxation. You can once again take some deep breaths into the lower abdomen and, now, add a rocking motion to the entire body, feeling yourself rock and sway like bamboo in the wind.

1. **Bring your feet closer together and place your hands over your lower abdomen.**

2. **Take a few deep breaths into the belly.**

3. **Relax into your body like bamboo in the wind, gently rocking back and forth or left and right.**

4. **Have the sense of being rooted and grounded through your legs but flexible through your body.**

5. **Rock and sway with your eyes closed for about 30 seconds. This rocking motion will allow your body to unwind and come back to a place of feeling centered.**

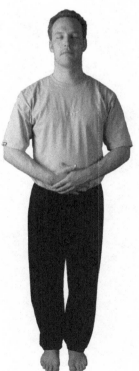

12

A Day of Magic

Your 7 Minutes of Magic routines and lifestyle suggestions can be used creatively to get the most out of your day. While the morning and evening routines will serve as the pillars of your day, you may find that some days allow you to do one routine and not the other. Do whatever your body needs. This program is designed to enhance your life in whatever ways your life allows. You can also incorporate the principles and other brief practices throughout the day to keep yourself centered and focused. The individual flows within each of the 7-minute routines can be used independently during the day when you need a little more energy or to clear a little stress.

A typical Day of Magic might look like this:

1. Wake up and practice 7 Minutes of Magic for the Morning.

2. Drink a large glass of water before you shower and get ready for work.

3. Have a light breakfast with green tea. For at least one bite of your breakfast, chew at least 20 times (preferably more, but

this is a good start) and set the intention that this food will energize your body for the day.

4. Take a mini-break in the late morning and practice the Wave breathing exercise (see pages 167–168), charging up the body with fresh oxygen.

5. Drink a large glass of water 20 minutes before lunch.

6. Again, during lunch, chew your food more thoroughly than you usually would, even if it is for just one bite.

7. Take a power nap early in the afternoon or practice the 7-Minute Meditation (see pages 153–154). For the nap, kick up your feet or lie on a couch or the floor. If you share an office, try going to a park or to your car to rest.

8. When you come home from work, greet your family, then ask them to give you a few minutes to change out of your work clothes. After changing, practice the 7 Minutes of Magic for the Evening.

9. Have a large glass of water 20 minutes before dinner.

10. While eating dinner, take time to chew your food thoroughly.

11. Take a 20-minute walk after dinner.

12. When you get into bed, take a moment to smile and to remember what you are grateful for in your life. Smiling and gratitude flood the body with positive hormones that heal and invigorate the entire system.

13. Just before going to sleep, practice the heart sound (see pages 158–159). Set your intention for a deep restful sleep.

Sometimes you can integrate all of these suggestions into your typical day; other times you are lucky if you drink a glass of water. Many people find it useful to photocopy this list as they are learning to incorporate these practices into their day.

Here are some other ways to integrate more magic into your daily life:

1. During your commute to and from work, practice deep breathing. Stoplights are especially good reminders to focus on your breath. Remember that deep breathing will greatly increase your energy and clear out stress.

2. If you are in a rush in the morning, just do the Energy Flow (pages 68–75), which stimulates your adrenal glands and wakes up your central nervous system like a quick caffeine shot of energy. It is well worth the 60 or 70 seconds. Your body will feel better, and your mind will be more focused.

3. Keep a large bottle of water at your desk or in your car and sip it throughout the day.

4. If you feel like someone or some situation is draining your energy, take 10 seconds and do the Centering movement (pages 179–180). This will allow you to experience more balance and greater calm.

5. If you are feeling tired at any point during the day, try doing a quick energy massage by knocking over the lower back area (see page 70). This is a natural way to stimulate adrenaline and energize the body.

6. If you have had an argument or a negative interaction with someone, try holding your hands out to the sides and mak-

ing the "Heeeee" sound (see pages 112–113). Remember, this sound was used at the end of the evening 7-minute routine for deep relaxation. It is also used to clear and let go of negative, stressful energy. Just take a deep breath and exhale, making the "Heeee" sound in a gentle whisper. Feel the negativity draining out of the body through your hands and feet.

7. Take time to smile and laugh throughout your day. Your body, heart, and mind will thank you.

Post this Magic Mirror reminder on a mirror in your home.

For your health, remember to do the 7 Minutes of Magic routines:

Breathe deeper.

Inhale into your lower abdomen, then your rib cage, then all the way into your chest.

Drink more water.

Drink an 8-ounce glass of water a half-hour before each meal and a total of eight glasses during the day.

Chew more, eat slower.

Chew each bite at least twenty times.

Meditate.

Breathe deeply, smile softly, and visualize golden light streaming through your body.

Enjoy your exercise.

Participate in fun activities three or four times a week for at least twenty minutes.

Do Tai Chi Walking.

Breathe deeply, inhaling and exhaling through the nose, and keep your mind focused in the present moment.

Spend time in nature.

Whether from a forest or a house plant, draw in nature's life-sustaining energy.

Take a power nap.

Find at least seven minutes to rejuvenate, but keep it to less than twenty minutes.

Calm your mind before you sleep.

Lying in bed, take a deep breath and exhale, making the heart sound softly ("Hawww").

Remember to smile and laugh.

Nothing is better for your health

Post this somewhere so you will see it every day as a reminder.

7 Minutes of Magic in the Morning

Core Flow

Upper Body Flow

Lower Body Flow

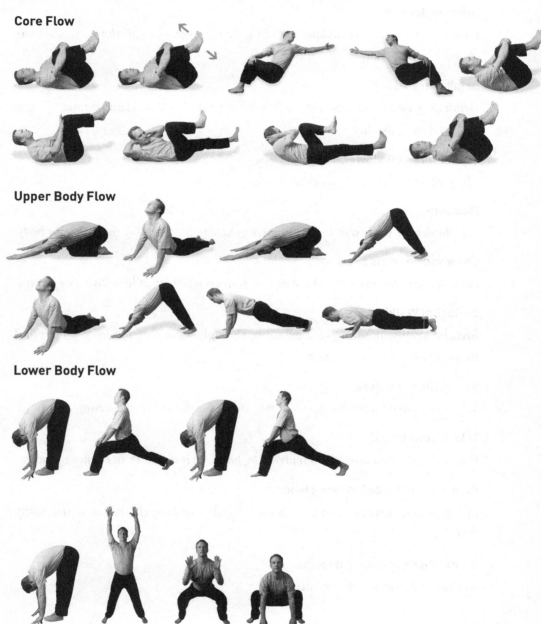

Post this somewhere where you can see it every day as a reminder.

7 Minutes of Magic in the Morning *(continued)*

Full Body Flow

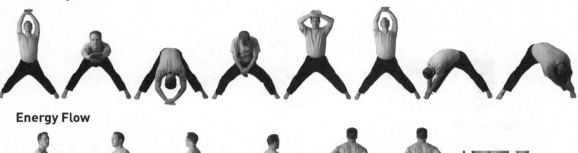

Energy Flow

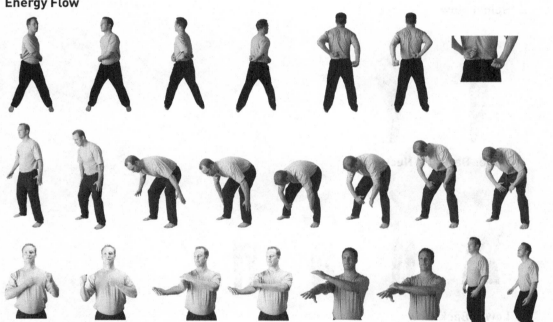

Breath Flow

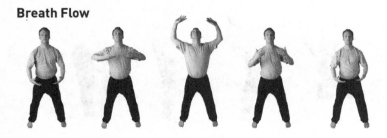

Post this somewhere where you can see it every day as a reminder.

7 Minutes of Magic in the Evening

Mind Flow

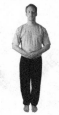

Spinal Flow

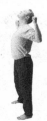 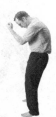

Upper Back and Neck Flow

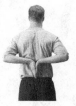 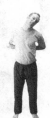 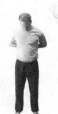 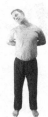

Lower Back Flow

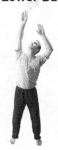 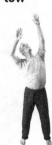 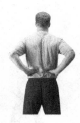 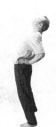 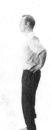 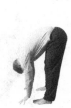

Post this somewhere where you can see it every day as a reminder.

7 Minutes of Magic in the Evening *(continued)*

Downward Flow

Seated Flow

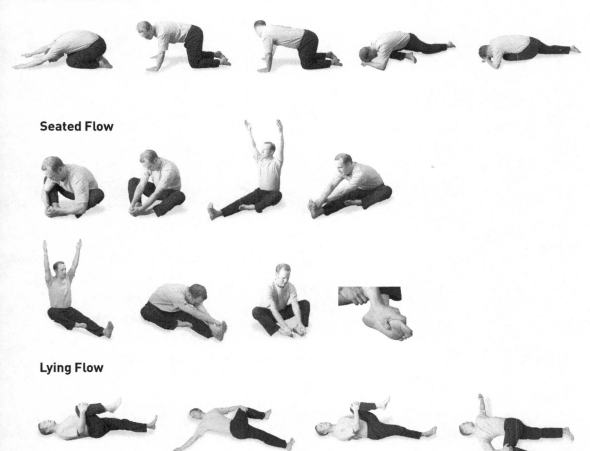

Lying Flow

Joy and Gratitude Flow

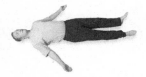

Index

Exercise to Heal

Discover the healing power of ancient methods of relaxation and meditiation, as seen on American Public Television and your local PBS station.

Find More "Magic" with Lee Holden!

Lee Holden is committed to creating simple, effective ways to bring your life into healthy balance, as with his breakthrough program 7 Minutes of Magic. Get even more out of your practice at www.ExerciseToHeal.com.

You'll find bonus information, video samples, and a new companion DVD, where Lee personally guides you through the 7 Minutes of Magic routine with expert tips and instructions, plus a bonus routine.

Visit www.ExerciseToHeal.com for a complete library of Lee's DVDs and CDs, all designed to keep you balanced, energized, and healthy. Through American Public Television, Lee's programs have aired on PBS stations nationwide.

About Lee Holden

Lee Holden is an internationally known instructor in meditation, tai chi, and qi gong. Lee's programs, through American Public Television, have reached millions of viewers in the United States and Canada. *Qi Gong for Beginners* with Lee Holden has aired on 105 PBS stations nationwide, reaching over 50 million households. Lee lectures and teaches workshops across the United States, as well as in Europe and Asia. Holden first discovered qi gong in his quest to achieve peak sports performance as a varsity soccer player at Berkeley. He later founded Pacific Healing Arts, one of northern California's most successful acupuncture and wellness centers. Lee has worked closely with Deepak Chopra, and serves as a stress management consultant to many corporations in Silicon Valley, including Apple and 3COM. He lives in California.

Printed in the United States
by Baker & Taylor Publisher Services

Printed in the United States
by Baker & Taylor Publisher Services